For more than twenty years Alice Miller taught and practised psychoanalysis. In 1973, due to her spontaneous painting she discovered her childhood history. She radically questioned the validity of psychoanalytic theories. As a result, in 1988 she resigned from the International Psychoanalytical Association and, in 1995, revised her bestselling *The Drama of Being a Child*.

Author of twelve books, which have been translated into thirty languages, Alice Miller has achieved worldwide recognition for her work on the causes and effects of child abuse, on violence towards children and its cost to society. She died in France in April 2010.

ALICE MILLER

The Drama of Being a Child

The Search for the True Self

Completely Revised and Updated
With a New Afterword by the Author

Translated by Ruth Ward

virago

VIRAGO

First published in Great Britain by Virago Press in 1987
Revised 2008

10

A previous version of chapter 1 appeared in the *International Journal of Psychoanalysis* 60 (1979), 47; a previous version of chapter 2 appeared in the *International Review of Psychoanalysis* 6 (1979), 61.

Grateful acknowledgment is made for permission to reprint excerpts from the following: Hermann Hesse, 'A Child's Heart,' from *Klinsoy's Last Summer*, translated by Richard and Clara Winston (New York: Farrar, Straus and Giroux, 1970, UK: Jonathan Cape), and *Damian,* translated by Michael Roloff and Michael Lebeck (New York: Harper & Row, 1965, UK: Peter Owen).

A CIP catalogue record for this book
is available from the British Library.

ISBN 978-1-86049-101-6

Typeset in Plantin by M Rules
Printed and bound in Great Britain by
Clays Ltd, St Ives plc

Papers used by Virago are from well-managed forests
and other responsible sources.

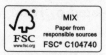

Virago
An imprint of
Little, Brown Book Group
Carmelite House
50 Victoria Embankment
London EC4Y 0DZ

An Hachette UK Company
www.hachette.co.uk

www.virago.co.uk

Contents

The Drama of Being a Child

1

The Drama of the Gifted Child and How We Became Psychotherapists

Experience has taught us that we have only one enduring weapon in our struggle against mental illness: the emotional discovery of the truth about the unique history of our childhood. Is it possible, then, to free ourselves altogether from illusions? History demonstrates that they sneak in everywhere, that every life is full of them – perhaps because the truth often seems unbearable to us. And yet the truth is so essential that its loss exacts a heavy toll, in the form of grave illness. In order to become whole we must try, in a long process, to discover our own personal truth, a truth that may cause pain before giving us a new sphere of freedom. If we choose instead to content ourselves with intellectual 'wisdom,' we will remain in the sphere of illusion and self-deception.

The damage done to us during our childhood cannot be undone, since we cannot change anything in our past. We can, however, change ourselves. We can repair ourselves and gain our lost integrity by choosing to look more closely at the knowledge that is stored inside our bodies and bringing this knowledge closer to our awareness. This path, although certainly not easy, is the only route by which we can at last leave behind the cruel, invisible prison of our childhood. We become free by transforming ourselves from unaware victims of the past into responsible individuals in the present, who are aware of our past and are thus able to live with it.

Most people do exactly the opposite. Without realizing that the past is constantly determining their present actions, they avoid learning anything about their history. They continue to live in their repressed childhood situation, ignoring the fact that it no longer exists. They are continuing to fear and avoid dangers that, although once real, have not been real for a long time. They are driven by unconscious memories and by repressed feelings and needs that determine nearly everything they do or fail to do.

The repression of brutal abuse experienced during

childhood drives many people to destroy their lives and the lives of others. In an unconscious thirst for revenge, they may engage in acts of violence, burning homes and businesses and physically attacking other people, using this destruction to hide the truth from themselves and avoid feeling the despair of the tormented child they once were. Such acts are often done in the name of 'patriotism' or religious beliefs.

Other people actively continue the torture once inflicted upon them in self-scourging clubs of every sort and in sado-masochistic practices. They think of such activities as 'liberation.' Women who allow their nipples to be pierced in order to hang rings from them can then pose for newspaper photographs, proudly saying that they felt no pain when having it done and that it was even fun for them. One need not doubt the truth of their statements; they had to learn very early in life not to feel pain, and today they would go to any lengths not to feel the pain of the little girl who was once sexually exploited by her father and had to imagine that it was fun for her.

Repressed pain may reveal itself more privately, as in a woman, sexually exploited as a child, who has denied her childhood reality and in order not to feel the pain is perpetually fleeing her past with the help of men, alcohol, drugs, or achievement. She needs a constant thrill to keep boredom at bay; not even one moment of quiet can be permitted during which the burning loneliness of her childhood experience might be felt, for she fears that feeling more than death. She will continue in her flight unless she learns that the awareness of old feelings is not deadly but liberating.

The repression of childhood pain influences not only the life of an individual but also the taboos of the whole society. The usual run of biographies illustrates this very clearly. In reading the biographies of famous artists, for example, one gains the impression that their lives began at puberty. Before that, we are told, they had a 'happy,' 'contented,' or 'untroubled' childhood, or one that was 'full of deprivation' or 'very stimulating.' But what a particular childhood really was like does not seem to interest these biographers – as if the roots of a whole life were not hidden and entwined in its childhood. I should like to illustrate this with a simple example.

Henry Moore describes in his memoirs how, as a small boy, he massaged his mother's back with an oil to soothe her rheumatism. Reading this suddenly threw light for me on Moore's sculptures: the great, reclining women with the tiny heads – I could now see in them the mother through the small boy's eyes, with the head high above, in diminishing perspective, and the back close before him and enormously enlarged. This interpretation may be irrelevant for many art critics, but for me it demonstrates how strongly a child's experiences may endure in his unconscious and what possibilities of expression they may awaken in the adult who is free to give them rein. Now, Moore's memory did not concern a traumatic event and so could survive intact. But every childhood's traumatic experiences remain hidden and locked in darkness, and the key to our understanding of the life that follows is hidden away with them.

THE POOR RICH CHILD

I sometimes ask myself whether it will ever be possible for us to grasp the extent of the loneliness and desertion to which we were exposed as children. Here I do not mean to speak, primarily, of children who were obviously uncared for or totally neglected, and who were always aware of this or at least grew up with the knowledge that it was so. Apart from these extreme cases, there are large numbers of people who enter therapy in the belief (with which they grew up) that their childhood was happy and protected.

Quite often I have been faced with people who were praised and admired for their talents and their achievements, who were toilet-trained in the first year of their lives, and who may even, at the age of one and a half to five, have capably helped to take care of their younger siblings. According to prevailing attitudes, these people – the pride of their parents – should have had a strong and stable sense of self-assurance. But the case is exactly the opposite. They do well, even excellently,

5

in everything they undertake; they are admired and envied; they are successful whenever they care to be – but behind all this lurks depression, a feeling of emptiness and self-alienation, and a sense that their life has no meaning. These dark feelings will come to the fore as soon as the drug of grandiosity fails, as soon as they are not 'on top,' not definitely the 'superstar,' or whenever they suddenly get the feeling they have failed to live up to some ideal image or have not measured up to some standard. Then they are plagued by anxiety or deep feelings of guilt and shame. What are the reasons for such disturbances in these competent, accomplished people?

In the very first interview they will let the listener know that they have had understanding parents, or at least one such, and if they are aware of having been misunderstood as children, they feel that the fault lay with them and with their inability to express themselves appropriately. They recount their earliest memories without any sympathy for the child they once were, and this is the more striking as these patients not only have a pronounced introspective ability but seem, to some degree, to be able to empathize with other people. Their access to the emotional world of their own childhood, however, is impaired – characterized by a lack of respect, a compulsion to control and manipulate, and a demand for achievement. Very often they show disdain and irony, even derision and cynicism, for

6

the child they were. In general, there is a complete absence of real emotional understanding or serious appreciation of their own childhood vicissitudes, and no conception of their true needs – beyond the desire for achievement. The repression of their real history has been so complete that their illusion of a good childhood can be maintained with ease.

As a basis for a description of the psychic climate of these persons, some general assumptions should be made clear:

- The child has a primary need from the very beginning of her life to be regarded and respected as the person she really is at any given time.
- When we speak here of 'the person she really is at any given time,' we mean emotions, sensations, and their expression from the first day onward.
- In an atmosphere of respect and tolerance for her feelings, the child, in the phase of separation, will be able to give up symbiosis with the mother and accomplish the steps toward individuation and autonomy.
- If they are to furnish these prerequisites for the healthy development of their child, the parents themselves ought to have grown up in such an atmosphere. If they did, they will be able to assure the child the protection and well-being she needs to develop trust.

- Parents who did not experience this climate as children are themselves deprived; throughout their lives they will continue to look for what their own parents could not give them at the appropriate time – the presence of a person who is completely aware of them and takes them seriously.

- This search, of course, can never fully succeed, since it relates to a situation that belongs irrevocably to the past, namely to the time right after birth and during early childhood.

- A person with this unsatisfied and unconscious (because repressed) need will nevertheless be compelled to attempt its gratification through substitute means, as long as she ignores her repressed life history.

- The most efficacious objects for substitute gratification are a parent's *own children*. The newborn baby or small child is completely dependent on his parents, and since their caring is essential for his existence, he does all he can to avoid losing them. From the very first day onward, he will muster all his resources to this end, like a small plant that turns toward the sun in order to survive.

In my work with people in the helping professions, I have often been confronted with a childhood history that seems significant to me.

- There was a *mother*⋆ who at the core was emotionally insecure and who depended for her equilibrium on her child's behaving in a particular way. This mother was able to hide her insecurity from her child and from everyone else behind a hard, authoritarian, even totalitarian facade.
- This child had an amazing ability to perceive and respond intuitively, that is, unconsciously, to this need of the mother, or of both parents, for him to take on the role that had unconsciously been assigned to him.
- This role secured 'love' for the child – that is, his parents' exploitation. He could sense that he was needed, and this need guaranteed him a measure of existential security.

This ability is then extended and perfected. Later, these children not only become mothers (confidantes, comforters, advisers, supporters) of their own mothers but also take over at least part of the responsibility for their siblings and eventually develop a special sensitivity to unconscious signals manifesting the needs of others. No wonder they often choose to become psychotherapists later on. Who else, without this previous history,

⋆By 'mother' I here refer to the person closest to the child during the first years of life. This need not be the biological mother, or even a woman. In the course of the past twenty years, many fathers have assumed this mothering function (Mütterlichkeit).

would muster sufficient interest to spend the whole day trying to discover what is happening in other people's unconscious? But the development and perfecting of this sensitivity – which once assisted the child in surviving and now enables the adult to pursue his strange profession – also contain the roots of his emotional disturbance: As long as the therapist is not aware of his repression, it can compel him to use his patients, who depend on him, to meet his unmet needs with substitutes.

THE LOST WORLD OF FEELINGS

On the basis of my experience, I think that the cause of an emotional disturbance is to be found in the infant's early adaptation. The child's needs for respect, echoing, understanding, sympathy, and mirroring have had to be repressed, with several serious consequences.

One such consequence is the person's inability to experience consciously certain feelings of his own (such as jealousy, envy, anger, loneliness, helplessness, or anxiety), either in childhood or later in adulthood. This is all the more tragic in that we are concerned here with lively people who are often capable of deep feelings. It is most noticeable when they describe childhood experiences that were free of pain and fear. They could enjoy their encounters with nature, for example, without hurting the mother or making her feel insecure, reducing her power, or endangering her equilibrium. It is remarkable how these attentive, lively, and sensitive children, who can, for example, remember exactly how they discovered the sunlight in bright grass at the age of four, at eight were unable to 'notice anything' or show any curiosity about their pregnant mother, or were 'not at all' jealous at the birth of a sibling. It is also remarkable how, at the age of two, such a child could be left alone and 'be good' while soldiers forced their way into the house and searched it, suffering the terrifying intrusion quietly and without crying. These people have all developed the art of not experiencing feelings, for a child can experience her feelings only when there is somebody there who accepts her fully, understands her, and supports her. If that person is missing, if the child must risk losing the mother's love or the love of her substitute in order to feel, then she will repress her emotions. She cannot even experience them secretly, 'just for herself'; she will fail to experience them at all. But they will nevertheless stay in her body, in her cells, stored up as information that can be triggered by a later event.

Throughout their later life, these people will have to deal with situations in which these rudimentary feelings may awaken, but without the original connection ever becoming clear. The connection can be deciphered only when the intense emotions have been experienced in therapy and successfully linked with their original situation.*

Take, for example, the feeling of abandonment – not that of the adult, who feels lonely and therefore turns to alcohol or drugs, goes to the movies, visits friends, or makes 'unnecessary' telephone calls in order to bridge the gap somehow. No, I mean the original feeling in the small infant, who had none of these means of distraction and whose communication, verbal or preverbal, did not reach the mother because his mother herself was deprived. For her part, she was dependent on a specific echo from the child that was essential to her, for she herself was a child in search of a person who could be available to her.

However paradoxical this may seem, a child is at the mother's disposal. The mother can feel herself the center of attention, for her child's eyes follow her every-where. A child cannot run away from her as her own mother once did. A child can be brought up so that it becomes what she wants it to be. A child can be made to show respect; she can impose her own feelings on him, see herself mirrored in his love and admiration, and feel strong in his presence. But when he becomes too much, she can abandon that child to a stranger or to solitary confinement in another room.

*In some new therapy methods, this phenomenon plays an essential role.

When a woman has had to repress all these needs in relation to her own mother, they will arise from the depth of her unconscious and seek gratification through her own child, however well-educated she may be. The child feels this clearly and very soon forgoes the expression of his own distress. Later, when these feelings of being deserted begin to emerge in the therapy of the adult, they are accompanied by intense pain and despair. It is clear that these people could not have survived so much pain as children. That would have been possible only in an empathic, attentive environment, which was lacking. Thus all feelings had to be warded off. But to say that they were *absent* would be a denial of the empirical evidence.

Several mechanisms can be recognized in the defense against early feelings of abandonment. In addition to simple denial, we usually find the exhausting struggle to fulfill the old, repressed, and by now often perverted needs with the help of symbols (cults, sexual perversions, groups of all kinds, alcohol, or drugs). Intellectualization is very commonly encountered as well, since it is a defense mechanism of great power. It can have disastrous results, however, when the mind ignores the vital messages of the body (see my reflections on Nietzsche's illness in *The Untouched Key* [1990] and *Breaking Down the Wall of Silence* [1991]). All these defense mechanisms are accompanied by repression of the original situation and the emotions belonging to it.

Accommodation to parental needs often (but not always) leads to the 'as-if personality.' This person develops in such a way that he reveals only what is expected of him and fuses so completely with what he reveals that one could scarcely guess how much more there is to him behind this false self. He cannot develop and differentiate his true self, because he is unable to live it. Understandably, this person will complain of a sense of emptiness, futility, or homelessness, for the emptiness is real. A process of emptying, impoverishment, and crippling of his potential actually took place. The integrity of the child was injured when all that was alive and spontaneous in him was cut off. In childhood, these patients have often had dreams in which they experienced themselves as at least partly dead. A young woman, Lisa, reported a recurrent dream:

> My younger siblings are standing on a bridge and throw a box into the river. I know that I am lying in it, dead, and yet I hear my heart beating; at this moment I always wake.

This dream combined her unconscious rage toward her younger siblings, for whom Lisa always had to be a loving, caring mother, with 'killing' her own feelings, wishes, and demands. A young man, Bob, dreamed:

> I see a green meadow, on which there is a white coffin. I am afraid that my mother is in it, but I open the lid and, luckily, it is not my mother but me.

If Bob had been able as a child to express his disappointment with his mother – to experience his rage and anger – he could have stayed fully alive. But that would have led to the loss of his mother's love, and that, for a child, can mean the same as death. So he 'killed' his anger, and with it a part of himself, in order to preserve the love of his mother. A young girl used to dream:

> I am lying on my bed. I am dead. My parents are talking and looking at me but they don't realize that I am dead.

The difficulties inherent in experiencing and developing one's own emotions lead to mutual dependency, which prevents individuation. Both parties have an interest in bond permanence. The parents have found in their child's false self the confirmation they were looking for, a substitute for their own missing security; the child, who has been unable to build up his own sense of security, is first consciously and then unconsciously dependent on his parents. He cannot rely on his own emotions, has not come to experience them through trial and error, has no sense of his own real needs, and is alienated from himself to the highest degree. Under these circumstances he cannot separate from his parents, and even as an adult he is still dependent on affirmation from his partner, from groups, and especially from his own children. The legacy of the parents is yet another generation condemned to hide from the true self while operating unconsciously under the influence of repressed memories. Unless the heir casts off his 'inheritance' by becoming fully conscious of his true past, and thus of his true nature, loneliness in the parental home will necessarily be followed by an adulthood lived in emotional isolation.

IN SEARCH OF THE TRUE SELF

How can therapy be of help here? It cannot give us back our lost childhood, nor can it change the past facts. No one can heal by maintaining or fostering illusion. The paradise of preambivalent harmony, for which so many patients hope, is unattainable. But the experience of one's own truth, and the postambivalent knowledge of it, make it possible to return to one's own world of feelings at an adult level – without paradise, but with the ability to mourn. And this ability does, indeed, give us back our vitality.

It is one of the turning points in therapy when the

patient comes to the emotional insight that all the love she has captured with so much effort and self-denial was not meant for her as she really was, that the admiration for her beauty and achievements was aimed at this beauty and these achievements and not at the child herself. In therapy, the small and lonely child that is hidden behind her achievements wakes up and asks: 'What would have happened if I had appeared before you sad, needy, angry, furious? Where would your love have been then? And I was all these things as well. Does this mean that it was not really me you loved, but only what I pretended to be? The well-behaved, reliable, empathic, understanding, and convenient child, who in fact was never a child at all? What became of my childhood? Have I not been cheated out of it? I can never return to it. I can never make up for it. From the beginning I have been a little adult. My abilities – were they simply misused?'

These questions are accompanied by much grief and pain, but the result is always a new authority that is establishing itself in the patient – a new empathy with her own fate, born out of mourning. Now the patient does not make light of manifestations of her self anymore, does not so often laugh or jeer at them, even if she still unconsciously passes them over or ignores them, in the same subtle way that her parents dealt with the child before she had any words to express her needs. Even as an older child, she was not allowed to

17

say, or even to think: 'I can be sad or happy whenever anything makes me sad or happy; I don't have to look cheerful for someone else, and I don't have to suppress my distress or anxiety to fit other people's needs. I can be angry and no one will die or get a headache because of it. I can rage when you hurt me, without losing you.'

In the majority of cases, it is a great relief to a patient to see that she can now recognize and take seriously the things she used to choke off, even if the old patterns come back, again and again, over a long period. But now she begins to understand that this strategy was her only chance to survive. Now she can *realize* how she still sometimes tries to persuade herself, when she is scared, that she is not; how she belittles her feelings to protect herself, and either does not become aware of them at all, or does so only several days after they have already passed. Gradually, she realizes how she is forced to look for distraction when she is moved, upset, or sad. (When a six-year-old's mother died, his aunt told him: 'You must be brave; don't cry; now go to your room and play nicely.')

Once the therapeutic process has started, it will continue if it is not interrupted by interpretations or other types of intellectual defense. The suffering person begins to be articulate and breaks with her former compliant attitudes, but because of her early experience she cannot believe she is not incurring mortal danger; she fears rejection and punishment when she defends her rights in the present. The patient is surprised by feelings she would rather not have recognized, but now it is too late: Awareness of her own impulses has already been aroused, and there is no going back.

Now the once intimidated and silenced child can experience herself in a way she had never before thought possible, and afterward she can enjoy the relief of having taken the risk and been true to herself. Whereas she had always despised miserliness, she suddenly catches herself counting up the two minutes lost to her session through a telephone call. Whereas she had previously never made demands herself and had always been tireless in fulfilling the demands of others, now she is suddenly furious that her therapist is again going on vacation. Or she is annoyed to see other people waiting outside the consulting room. What can this be? Surely not jealousy. That is an emotion she does not know! And yet: 'What are they doing here? Do others besides me come here?' She hadn't realized that before.

At first it will be mortifying to see that she is not always good, understanding, tolerant, controlled, and, above all, without needs, for these have been the basis of her self-respect.

There is a big difference between having ambivalent feelings toward someone as an adult and suddenly experiencing oneself as a two-year-old being fed by the maid in the kitchen and thinking in despair: 'Why does

Mom go out every evening? Why does she not take pleasure in me? What is wrong with me that she prefers to go to other people? What can I do to make her stay home? Just don't cry, just don't cry.' Peter as a two-year-old child could not have thought in these words, but in the therapeutic session where he experienced this reality, he was both an adult and a toddler, and could cry bitterly. It was not a cathartic crying, but rather the integration of his earlier longing for his mother, which until now he had always denied. In the following weeks Peter went through all the torments of his ambivalence toward his mother, who was a successful pediatrician. Her previously 'frozen,' idealized portrait melted into the picture of a woman who had not been able to give her child any continuity in their relationship. 'I hated those beasts who were constantly sick and always taking you away from me. I hated you because you preferred being with them to being with me.' Feelings of helplessness were mingled with long-dammed-up rage against the mother who had not been available to him when he needed her the most. As a result of becoming aware of these feelings, Peter could rid himself of a symptom that had tormented him for a long time; its point was now easy to understand. His relationships to women changed as his compulsion first to conquer and then to desert them disappeared.

Peter experienced his early feelings of helplessness, of anger, and of being at the mercy of his mostly absent mother in a manner that he could not previously have remembered. One can only remember what has been consciously experienced. But the emotional world of a tormented child is itself the result of a selective process that has eliminated the most important elements. These early feelings, joined with the pain of being unable to understand what is going on – which is part of the earliest period of childhood – are consciously experienced for the first time during therapy.

It is like a miracle each time to see how much authenticity and integrity have survived behind dissimulation, denial, and self-alienation, and how they can reappear as soon as the patient finds access to the feelings. Nevertheless, it would be wrong to imply that there is a fully developed, true self consciously hidden behind the false self. The important point is that the child does not know what he is hiding. Karl, age forty-two, expressed this in the following way:

> I lived in a glass house into which my mother could look at any time. In a glass house, however, you cannot conceal anything without giving yourself away, except by hiding it under the ground. And then you cannot see it yourself, either.

An adult can be fully aware of his feelings only if he had caring parents or caregivers. People who were abused and neglected in childhood are missing this capacity and are therefore never overtaken by unex-pected emotions. They will admit only those feelings that are accepted and approved by their inner censor, who is their parents' heir. Depression and a sense of inner emptiness are the price they must pay for this control. The true self cannot communicate because it has remained unconscious, and therefore undeveloped, in its inner prison. The company of prison warders does not encourage lively development. It is only after it is liberated that the self begins to be articulate, to grow, and to develop its creativity. Where there had been only fearful emptiness or equally frightening grandiose fan-tasies, an unexpected wealth of vitality is now discovered. This is not a homecoming, since this home has never before existed. It is the creation of home.

THE THERAPIST'S HISTORY

It is often said that psychotherapists suffer from an emotional disturbance. My purpose so far has been to clarify the extent to which this assertion can be shown to have a basis in experience. The therapist's sensibility, empathy, responsiveness, and powerful 'antennae' indi-cate that as a child he probably used to fulfill other people's needs and to repress his own.

Of course, there is the theoretical possibility that a sensitive child could have had parents who did not need to misuse him – parents who saw him as he really was, understood him, and tolerated and respected his feelings. Although such a child would develop a healthy sense of security, one could hardly expect that he would later take up the profession of psychotherapy; that he would cultivate and develop his sensitivity to others to the same extent as those whose parents used them to gratify their own needs; and that he would ever be able to understand sufficiently – without the basis of experience – what it means to 'have killed' one's self.

I think that our childhood fate can indeed enable us to practice psychotherapy, but only if we have been given the chance, through our own therapy, to live with the reality of our past and to give up the most flagrant of our illusions. This means tolerating the knowledge that, to avoid losing the 'love' of our parents, we were compelled to gratify their unconscious needs at the cost of our own emotional development. It also means being able to experience the resentment and mourning aroused by our parents' failure to fulfill our primary needs. If we have never consciously lived through this despair and the resulting rage, and have therefore never been able to work through it, we will be in danger of transferring this situation, which then would remain unconscious, onto our patients. It would not be surprising if our unconscious need should find no better way than to make use of a weaker person. Most readily available for exploitation are one's own children or one's patients, who at times are as obedient and as dependent on their therapists as children are on their parents.

A patient with 'antennae' for his therapist's unconscious will react promptly. If he senses that it is important to his therapist to have patients who soon become autonomous and behave with self-confidence, he will quickly feel himself autonomous and react accordingly. He can do that; he can do anything that is expected of him. But because this autonomy is not genuine, it soon ends in depression. True autonomy is preceded by the experience of being dependent. True liberation can be found only beyond the deep ambivalence of infantile dependence.

When he presents material that fits the therapist's knowledge, concepts, and skills – and therefore also his expectations – the patient satisfies his therapist's wish for approval, echo, understanding, and for being taken seriously. In this way the therapist exercises the same sort of unconscious manipulation as that to which he was exposed as a child. A child can never see through *unconscious manipulation*. It is like the air he breathes; he knows no other, and it appears to him to be the only breathable air.

What happens if we don't recognize the harmful quality of this air, even in adulthood? We will pass this harm on to others, while pretending that we are acting only for their own good. The more insight I gain into the unconscious manipulation of children by their parents, the more urgent it seems to me that we resolve our repression. Not only as parents but also as therapists, we must be willing to face our history. Only after painfully experiencing and accepting our own truth can we be free from the hope that we might still find an understanding, empathic 'parent' – perhaps in a patient – who will be at our disposal.

This temptation to seek a parent among our patients should not be underestimated; our own parents seldom or never listened to us with such rapt attention as our patients usually do, and they never revealed their inner world to us as clearly and honestly as do our patients at times. Only the never-ending work of mourning can help us from lapsing into the illusion that we have found the parent we once urgently needed – empathic and open, understanding and understandable, honest and available, helpful and loving, feeling, transparent, clear, without unintelligible contradictions. Such a parent was never ours, for a mother can react empathically only to the extent that she has become free of her own childhood; when she denies the vicissitudes of her early life, she wears invisible chains.

Children who are intelligent, alert, attentive, sensitive, and completely attuned to the mother's well-being are entirely at her disposal. Transparent, clear, and reliable, they are easy to manipulate as long as their true self (their emotional world) remains in the cellar of the glass house in which they have to live – sometimes until puberty or until they come to therapy, and very often until they have become parents themselves.

Robert, now thirty-one, could never be sad or cry as a child, without being aware that he was making his beloved mother unhappy and very unsure of herself. The extremely sensitive child felt himself warded off by his mother, who had been in a concentration camp as a child but had never spoken about it. Not until her son was grown up and could ask her questions did she tell him that she had been one of eighty children who had had to watch their parents going into the gas chambers and that not one child had cried. Because 'cheerfulness' was the trait that had saved her life in childhood, her own children's tears threatened her equilibrium. Throughout his childhood this son had tried to be cheerful. He could express glimpses of his true self and his feelings only in obsessive perversions, which seemed alien, shameful, and incomprehensible to him until he began to grasp their real meaning.

One is totally defenseless against this sort of manipulation in childhood. The tragedy is that the parents too have no defense against it, as long as they refuse to face their own history. If the repression stays unresolved, the parents' childhood tragedy is unconsciously continued on in their children.

Another example may illustrate this more clearly. A father who as a child had often been frightened by the anxiety attacks of his periodically schizophrenic mother

26

and was never given an explanation enjoyed telling his beloved small daughter gruesome stories. He always laughed at her fears and afterward comforted her with the words: 'But it is only a made-up story. You don't need to be scared, you are here with me.' In this way he could manipulate his child's fear and have the feeling of being strong. His conscious wish was to give the child something valuable of which he himself had been deprived, namely protection, comfort, and explanations. But what he unconsciously handed on was his own childhood fear, the expectation of disaster, and the unanswered question (also from his childhood): Why does this person I love frighten me so much?

Probably everybody has a more or less concealed inner chamber that she hides even from herself and in which the props of her childhood drama are to be found. Those who will be most affected by the contents of this hidden chamber are her children. When the mother was a child she hardly had a chance to understand what happened; she could only develop symptoms. As an adult in therapy, however, she can resolve these symptoms if she allows herself to feel what they were able to disguise: feelings of horror, indignation, despair, and helpless rage.

Can it be an accident that Heinrich Pestalozzi – who was fatherless from his sixth year onward and emotionally neglected despite the presence of his mother and of a nurse – neglected his only son, although he was capable, on the other hand, of giving orphan children genuine warmth and fatherliness? This son was finally considered to be mentally defective, although he had been an intelligent child.* He died at the age of thirty. Both his life and his death caused Pestalozzi much pain and guilt (Ganz, 1966, Lavater-Sloman, 1977). It was also Pestalozzi who is reputed to have said: 'You can drive the devil out of your garden but you will find him again in the garden of your son.'

THE GOLDEN BRAIN

Alphonse Daudet's *Lettres de mon Moulin* includes a story that may sound rather bizarre but nevertheless has much in common with what I have presented here. I shall summarize the story briefly:

> Once upon a time there was a child who had a golden brain. His parents only discovered this by chance when he injured his head and gold instead

---

*In H. Ganz (1966) we can read: 'On the occasion of his father's nameday, the five-year-old Jakobli, who could not write, . . . gaily dictated to his mother: "I wish my dear Papa . . . that you should see a lot more and I thank you a hundred thousand times for your goodness . . . that you have brought me up so joyfully and lovingly. Now I shall speak from my heart. . . . It makes me terribly happy, if you can say: I have brought my son up to happiness. . . . I am his joy and his happiness. Then shall I first give thanks for what you have done in my life. . . ."' (p. 53) of blood flowed out. They then began to look after him carefully and would not let him play with other children for fear of being robbed. When the boy was grown up and wanted to go out into the world, his mother said: 'We have done so much for you, we ought to be able to share your wealth.' Then her son took a large piece of gold out of his brain and gave it to his mother. He lived in great style with a friend who, however, robbed him one night and ran away. After that the man resolved to guard his secret and to go out to work, because his reserves were visibly dwindling. One day he fell in love with a beautiful girl who loved him too, but no more than the beautiful clothes he gave her so lavishly. He married her and was very happy, but after two years she died and he spent the rest of his wealth on her funeral, which had to be splendid. Once, as he was creeping through the streets, weak, poor, and unhappy, he saw a beautiful little pair of boots that would have been perfect for his wife. He forgot that she was dead – perhaps because his emptied brain no longer worked – and entered the shop to buy the boots. But in that very moment he fell, and the shopkeeper saw a dead man lying on the ground.

Daudet, who was to die from an illness of the spinal cord, wrote following this story:

This story sounds as though it were invented, but it is true from beginning to end. There are people who have to pay for the smallest things in life with their very substance and their spinal cord. That is a constantly recurring pain, and then when they are tired of suffering . . .

Does not mother love belong to the 'smallest,' but also indispensable, things in life, for which many people paradoxically have to pay by giving up their living selves?

2

Depression and Grandiosity: Two Related Forms of Denial

THE VICISSITUDES OF THE CHILD'S NEEDS

Every child has a legitimate need to be noticed, understood, taken seriously, and respected by his mother. In the first weeks and months of life he needs to have the mother at his disposal, must be able to avail himself of her and be mirrored by her. This is beautifully illustrated in one of Donald Winnicott's images: the mother gazes at the baby in her arms, and the baby gazes at his mother's face and finds himself therein . . . provided that the mother is really looking at the unique, small, helpless being and not projecting her own expectations, fears, and plans for the child. In that case, the child would find not himself in his mother's face, but rather the mother's own projections. This child would remain without a mirror, and for the rest of his life would be seeking this mirror in vain.

Healthy Development

If a child is lucky enough to grow up with a mirroring, available mother who is at the child's disposal – that is, a mother who allows herself to be made use of as a function of the child's development – then a healthy self-feeling can gradually develop in the growing child. Ideally, this mother should also provide the necessary emotional climate and understanding for the child's needs. But even a mother who is not especially warm-hearted can make this development possible, if only she refrains from preventing it and allows the child to acquire from other people what she herself lacks. Various studies have shown the incredible ability a child displays in making use of the smallest affective 'nourishment' (stimulation) to be found in his surroundings.

I understand a healthy self-feeling to mean the unquestioned certainty that the feelings and needs one experiences are a part of one's self. This certainty is not something one can gain upon reflection; it is there like one's own pulse, which one does not notice as long as it functions normally.

The automatic, natural contact with his own emotions and needs gives an individual strength and *self-esteem.* He may experience his feelings – sadness, despair, or the need for help – without fear of making the mother insecure. He can allow himself to be afraid when he is threatened, angry when his wishes are not fulfilled. He knows not only what he does not want but also what he wants and is able to express his wants, irrespective of whether he will be loved or hated for it.

If a woman is to give her child what he will need throughout his life, it is absolutely fundamental that she not be separated from her newborn, for the hormones that foster and nourish her motherly instinct are released immediately after birth and continue in the following days and weeks as she grows more familiar with her baby. When a newborn is separated from his mother – which was the rule not so long ago in maternity hospitals and still occurs in the majority of cases, out of ignorance and for the sake of convenience – then a great opportunity is missed for both mother and child.

The bonding (through skin and eye contact) between mother and baby after birth stimulates in both of them the feeling that they belong together, a feeling of oneness that ideally has been growing from the time of conception. The infant is given the sense of safety he needs to trust his mother, and the mother receives the instinctive reassurance that will help her understand and answer her child's messages. This initial mutual intimacy can never again be created, and its absence can be a serious obstacle right from the start.

The crucial significance of bonding has only recently been proved scientifically. One hopes that it will soon be taken into account in practice, not only in a few select maternity hospitals but in larger hospitals as well, so that everyone will benefit from it. A woman who has experienced bonding with her child will be in less danger of mistreating him and will be in a better position to protect him from mistreatment by the father and other caregivers, such as teachers and babysitters.

Even a woman whose own repressed history has been responsible for a lack of bonding with her child can later help him overcome this deficit, if she comes to understand its significance. She will also be able to compensate for the consequences of a difficult birth if she does not minimize their importance and knows that a child who was heavily traumatized at the beginning of his life will be in particular need of care and attention in order to overcome the fears arising out of more recent experiences.

The Disturbance

What happens if a mother not only is unable to recognize and fulfill her child's needs, but is herself in need of assurance? Quite unconsciously, the mother then tries to assuage her own needs through her child. This does not rule out strong affection; the mother often

34

loves her child passionately, but not in the way he needs to be loved. The reliability, continuity, and constancy that are so important for the child are therefore missing from this exploitative relationship. What is missing above all is the framework within which the child could experience his feelings and emotions. Instead, he develops something the mother needs, and although this certainly saves his life (by securing the mother's or the father's 'love') at the time, it may nevertheless prevent him, throughout his life, from being himself.

In such cases the natural needs appropriate to the child's age cannot be integrated, so they are repressed or split off. This person will later live in the past without realizing it and will continue to react to past dangers as if they were present.

People who have asked for my assistance because of their depression have usually had to deal with a mother who was extremely insecure and who often suffered from depression herself. The child, most often an only child or the first-born, was seen as the mother's possession. What the mother had once failed to find in her own mother she was able to find in her child: someone at her disposal who could be used as an echo and could be controlled, who was completely centered on her, would never desert her, and offered her full attention and admiration. If the child's demands became too great (as those of her own mother once did), she was no longer so defenseless: she could refuse to allow herself to be tyrannized; she could bring the child up in such a way that he neither cried nor disturbed her. At last she could make sure that she received consideration, care, and respect.

Barbara, a mother of four children, at thirty-five had only scanty memories of her childhood relationship with her mother. At the beginning of treatment, she described her as an affectionate, warmhearted woman who spoke to her 'openly about her own troubles' at an early age, who was very concerned for her children, and who sacrificed herself for her family. She was often asked for advice by others within the sect to which the family belonged. Barbara reported that her mother had always been especially proud of her. The mother was now old and an invalid, and the patient was very concerned about her health. She often dreamed that something had happened to her mother and woke up with great anxiety.

As a consequence of the emotions that arose in Barbara through therapy, this picture of her mother changed. Above all, when memories of toilet-training entered her consciousness, she experienced her mother as demanding, controlling, manipulative, cold, petty, obsessive, easily offended, and hard to please. Many subsequent childhood memories of her mother confirmed these characteristics. Barbara was then able to connect with the real reasons for her long-suppressed anger and to discover what her mother was really like. She realized that when her mother had felt insecure in relation to her, she had in fact often been cold and had treated her badly. The mother's anxious concern for the child had served to ward off her aggression and envy. Since the mother had often been humiliated as a child, she needed to be valued by her daughter.

Barbara experienced in therapy for the first time the agonizing fear and rage she had had to repress when she was ten years old and came home from school on her mother's birthday to find her lying on the floor with closed eyes. The child cried out, thinking her mother was dead. The mother then opened her eyes and said, delighted, 'You gave me the most precious birthday gift. Now I know that you love me, that somebody loves me.' For decades pity and compassion hindered Barbara from realizing the cruelty with which she had been treated. Triggered by a later event, this memory could finally emerge, accompanied by feelings of rage and indignation.

Gradually, the different pictures of the mother were united into that of a single human being whose weakness, insecurity, and oversensitivity made her do everything she could to keep her child at her disposal. The mother, who apparently functioned well with others, was herself basically still a child cut off from her real emotions. The daughter, on the other hand, took over the understanding and caring role until she discovered, with her own children, her previously ignored needs. Before she recognized the story of her past, she had been compelled to press her children into her service, as her mother had done.

THE ILLUSION OF LOVE

Over the years, my work has included many initial consultations with people whom I saw for one or two sessions before referring them to a colleague. In these short encounters, the tragedy of an individual history can often be seen with moving clarity. In what is described as depression and experienced as emptiness, futility, fear of impoverishment, and loneliness can usually be recognized as the tragic loss of the self in childhood, manifested as the total alienation from the self in the adult.

I have witnessed various mixtures and nuances of so-called narcissistic disturbances. For the sake of clarity, I shall describe two extreme forms, of which I consider one to be the reverse of the other – grandiosity and depression. Behind manifest grandiosity there constantly lurks depression, and behind a depressive mood there often hides an unconscious (or conscious but split off) sense of a tragic history. In fact, grandiosity is the defense against depression, and depression is the defense against the deep pain over the loss of the self that results from denial.

Grandiosity

The person who is 'grandiose' is admired everywhere and needs this admiration; indeed, he cannot live without it. He must excel brilliantly in everything he undertakes, which he is surely capable of doing (otherwise he just does not attempt it). He, too, admires himself, for his qualities – his beauty, cleverness, talents – and for his success and achievements. Beware if one of these fails him, for then the catastrophe of a severe depression is imminent.

It is usually considered normal when sick or aged people who have suffered the loss of much of their health and vitality or women who are experiencing menopause become depressive. There are, however, many people who can tolerate the loss of beauty, health, youth, or loved ones and, although they grieve, do so without depression. In contrast, there are those with great gifts, often precisely the most gifted, who do suffer from severe depression. For one is free from it only when self-esteem is based on the authenticity of one's own feelings and not on the possession of certain qualities.

The collapse of self-esteem in a 'grandiose' person will show clearly how precariously that self-esteem has been hanging in the air – 'hanging from a balloon,' as a patient once dreamed. That balloon flew up very high in a good wind but was suddenly punctured and soon lay like a little rag on the ground, for nothing genuine that could have given inner strength and support had ever been developed.

In a field study conducted at Chestnut Lodge, Maryland, in 1954, the family backgrounds of twelve patients suffering from manic-depressive psychoses were examined. The results strongly confirm the conclusions I have reached, by other means, about the etiology of depression:

> All the patients came from families who were socially isolated and felt themselves to be too little respected in their neighborhood. They therefore made special efforts to increase their prestige with their neighbors through conformity and outstanding achievements. The child who later became ill had been assigned a special role in this effort. He was supposed to guarantee the family honor, and was loved only in proportion to the degree to which he was able to fulfill the demands of this family ideal by *means of his special abilities, talents, his beauty, etc.** If he failed, he was punished by being cold-shouldered or thrown out of the family group, and by the knowledge that he had brought great shame on his people. (Eicke-Spengler 1977, p. 1104)

*Italics added.

With today's mobility of families and family members, adapting to a different ethnic culture is essential to survival, but it is threatening to the child's autonomy. Unfortunately, the only 'alternative' seems to be a clinging to, or return to, fundamentalism.

Without therapy, it is impossible for the grandiose person to cut the tragic link between admiration and love. He seeks insatiably for admiration, of which he never gets enough because admiration is not the same thing as love. It is only a substitute gratification of the primary needs for respect, understanding, and being taken seriously – needs that have remained unconscious since early childhood. Often a whole life is devoted to this substitute. As long as the true need is not felt and understood, the struggle for the symbol of love will continue. It is for this very reason that an aging, world-famous photographer who had received many international awards could say to an interviewer, 'I've never felt what I have done was good enough.' And he does not question why he has felt this way. Apparently, it has never occurred to him that the depression he reports could be related to his fusion with the demands of his parents.

A patient once spoke of the feeling of always having to walk on stilts. Is somebody who always has to walk on stilts not bound to be constantly envious of those who can walk on their own legs, even if they seem to him to be smaller and more 'ordinary' than he is himself? And is he not bound to carry pent-up rage within himself, against those who have made him afraid to walk without stilts? He could also be envious of healthy people because they do not have to make a constant effort to earn admiration, and because they do not have to do something in order to impress, one way or the other, but are free to be 'average.'

The grandiose person is never really free; first, because he is excessively dependent on admiration from others, and second, because his self-respect is dependent on qualities, functions, and achievements that can suddenly fail.

Depression as the Reverse of Grandiosity

In many of the patients I have known, depression was coupled with grandiosity in many ways.

1: Depression sometimes appeared when grandiosity *broke down* as a result of sickness, disablement, or aging. In the case of an unmarried woman, external sources of approval gradually dried up as she grew older. She no longer received constant confirmation of her attractiveness, which earlier had served a directly supportive function as a substitute for the missing mirroring by her mother. Superficially, her despair about getting old seemed to be due to the absence of sexual contacts but, at a deeper level, early fears of being abandoned were now aroused, and this woman had no new conquests with which to counteract them. All her substitute mirrors were broken. She again stood helpless and confused, as the small girl once did before her mother's face, in which she found not herself but only her mother's confusion.

Men often experience becoming older in a similar way, even if a new love affair may seem to create the illusion of their youth for a time and may in this way introduce brief manic phases into the early stages of the depression brought to the surface by their aging.

2: In the combination of *alternating phases* of grandiosity and depression, their common ground can be recognized. They are the two sides of a medal that can be described as the 'false self,' a medal that was once actually won for achievement.

For example, at the height of his success an actor can play before an enthusiastic audience and experience feelings of heavenly greatness and almightiness. Nevertheless, his sense of emptiness and futility, even of shame and anger, can return the next morning if his happiness the previous night was not only due to his creative activity in playing and expressing the part but was also, and above all, rooted in the substitute satisfaction of old needs for echoing, mirroring, and being seen and understood. If his success the previous night serves only to deny childhood frustrations, then, like every substitute, it can bring only momentary satisfaction. In fact, true satisfaction is no longer possible, since the right time for that now lies irrevocably in the past. The former child no longer exists, nor do the former parents. The present parents – if they are still alive – are now old and dependent; they no longer have any power over their son and are perhaps delighted with his success and with his infrequent visits. In the present, the son enjoys success and recognition, but these things cannot offer him more than their present value; they cannot fill the old gap. Again, as long as he is able to deny this need with the help of illusion – that is, with the intoxication of success – the old wound cannot heal. Depression leads him close to his wounds, but only mourning for what he has missed, *missed at the crucial time*, can lead to real healing.*

---

*Let me cite a remark by Igor Stravinsky as an example of successful mourning: 'I am convinced that it was my misfortune that my father was spiritually very distant from me and that even my mother had no love for me. When my oldest brother died unexpectedly (with my mother transferring her feelings from him onto me, and my father, also, remaining as reserved as ever), I resolved that one day I would show them, now this day has come and gone. No one remembers this day but me, who am its only remaining witness.' This is in marked contrast to a statement by Samuel Beckett: 'One could say that I had a happy childhood, although I showed little talent for being happy. My parents did all that can be done to make a child happy, but I often felt very lonely.' Beckett's childhood drama had been fully repressed, and idealization of the parents had been maintained with the help of denial, yet the boundless isolation of his childhood found expression in his plays. (For both quotations, see Mueller-Braunschweig, 1974.)

3: Continuous performance of outstanding achievements may sometimes enable a person to maintain the illusion of the constant attention and availability of his parents (whose absence from his early childhood he now denies just as thoroughly as his own emotional reactions). Such a person is usually able to ward off threatening depression with *increased displays of brilliance,* thereby deceiving both himself and those around him. However, he quite often chooses a marriage partner who either already has strong depressive traits or, at least within their marriage, unconsciously takes over and enacts the depressive components of the grandiose partner. The depression is thus kept outside, and the grandiose one can look after his 'poor' partner, protect her like a child, feel strong and indispensable, and thus gain another supporting pillar for the building of his own personality. Actually, however, that personality has no secure foundation and is dependent on the supporting pillars of success, achievement, 'strength,' and, above all, the denial of the emotional world of his childhood.

Although the outward picture of depression is quite the opposite of that of grandiosity and has a quality that expresses the tragedy of the loss of self in a more obvious way, they have many points in common:

- A false self that has led to the loss of the potential true self

45

- A fragility of self-esteem because of a lack of confidence in one's own feelings and wishes
- Perfectionism
- Denial of rejected feelings
- A preponderance of exploitative relationships
- An enormous fear of loss of love and therefore a great readiness to conform
- Split-off aggression
- Oversensitivity
- A readiness to feel shame and guilt
- Restlessness.

Depression as Denial of the Self

Depression consists of a denial of one's own emotional reactions. This denial begins in the service of an absolutely essential adaptation during childhood and indicates a very early injury. There are many children who have not been free, right from the beginning, to experience the very simplest of feelings, such as discontent, anger, rage, pain, even hunger – and, of course, enjoyment of their own bodies.

Beatrice, fifty-eight, the daughter of missionary parents and a sufferer of deep depression, never knew whether she was hungry or not. Her mother had written proudly in her diary that at the age of three months Beatrice had already learned to *wait* to be fed and to suppress her hunger, without crying. Discontent and anger aroused uncertainty in her mother, and her children's pain made her anxious. Her children's enjoyment of their bodies aroused both her envy and her shame about 'what other people would think.' Under such circumstances, a child may learn very early in life what she is not supposed to feel.

If we have thrown away the keys to understanding our lives, the causes of depression – as well as those of all suffering, illness, and healing – must remain a mystery to us, regardless of whether we call ourselves psychiatrists or authorities in the sciences or both. When psychiatrists with decades of experience have never dared to face their own reality and have instead spent their time (and their parents' time) talking about 'dysfunctional families,' they will need a concept like a 'Higher Power' or God to explain to themselves the 'miracle' of healing. They will then behave like people who are faithfully trying to follow a map, without realizing that the first step they took was in the wrong direction. Because they have lost the way from the very start, their 'scientific' fidelity to the map doesn't give them the expected results and doesn't take them where they want to go. I would like to illustrate this with an example.

A psychiatrist whose book was sent to me by a reader argues that mistreatment, neglect, and exploitation in childhood cannot be the only causes of psychic illnesses. There must, he feels, be other, irrational reasons that can explain why one person apparently escapes the catastrophic effects of abuse – or at least is able to heal more quickly – while another seems to suffer more intensely or for a longer time. It must, he suspects, be 'grace.'

He reports the story of a patient who lived with his single mother in extreme poverty for the first year of his life and who was then taken away from her by the authorities. He was placed in one foster home after another, and in all of them the child was severely mistreated. But when he became a psychiatric patient, he healed faster than many others with less obvious stories of abuse. How could this man, who had endured unspeakable cruelty in his childhood and youth, liberate himself so readily from his symptoms? Was it with God's help?

Many people love this type of explanation, without raising a very significant question: Shouldn't we ask why God was willing neither to help other patients of this psychiatrist nor to help this man when he was being beaten mercilessly as a child? Was it really God's grace that helped him as an adult, or is the explanation more prosaic? If this man had a mother who, in spite of her poverty, gave him real love, respect, protection, and security in his first year, he would have had a better start in life and would then have been better able to deal with later abuse than would a patient whose integrity was injured from the first day of her life – as was Beatrice, for instance.

Beatrice was not physically mistreated in her youth. She did, however, have to learn as a small infant how to make her mother happy by not crying, by not being hungry – by not having any needs at all. She suffered first from anorexia and then, throughout her adult life, from severe depression. Psychiatrists are denying this type of damage when they talk about 'grace' and other 'spiritual' qualities. In order to acknowledge the consequences of such early, hidden trauma, they would first have to do some hard work on themselves. Once they become willing to face the facts – their *own* facts – they will lose interest in teaching others about grace and other 'mysteries' in the name of science.

Clinging uncritically to traditional ideas and beliefs often serves to obscure or deny real facts of our life history. Without free access to these facts, the sources of our ability to love remain cut off. No wonder, then, that even well-intended moral appeals – to be loving, caring, generous, and so forth – are fruitless. We cannot really love if we are forbidden to know our truth, the truth about our parents and caregivers as well as about ourselves. We can only try *to behave as if we were loving*. But this hypocritical behavior is the opposite of love. It is confusing and deceptive, and it produces much helpless rage in the deceived person. This rage must be repressed in the presence of the pretended 'love,' especially if one is dependent, as a child is, on the person who is masquerading in this illusion of love.

We could make great progress in becoming more honest, respectful, and conscious, thus less destructive, if religious leaders could acknowledge and respect these simple psychological laws. Instead of ignoring them, they should open their eyes to the vast damage produced by hypocrisy, in families and in society as a whole. Vera's letter to me, from which she asked me to quote, gives a clear example of this confusion and damage. And Maja's history shows how spontaneous love for a child eventually became possible for her, once the repression of her past had been resolved. Vera, age fifty-two, wrote:

I had been a chronic alcoholic since adolescence, and I finally became sober thanks to Alcoholics Anonymous. I was so grateful for this liberation from my alcohol addiction that I attended every weekly meeting for eleven years. For a long time I managed to ignore and override my own critical thoughts concerning the moral issues represented there. I even succeeded at first in not taking any notice of the serious illness I began to develop (eventually diagnosed as multiple sclerosis) and in making light of the symptoms. It was only when my depressive moods became longer and refused to disappear that I began to face my truth.

It was very hard at first. When I succeeded in retrieving some repressed memories, they were close to unbearable. I wanted to stop. But my curiosity and my pain were stronger than my fear, and I decided to continue. During the first year of intensive work some of my symptoms disappeared. Now, after three years of work with this method, I understand that these symptoms *had* to develop in order to wake me from my dangerous sleep so that I could finally take seriously my feelings, perceptions, and thoughts.

I knew, for instance, that I had often become angry when 'unconditional love' was discussed in the group meetings. I was apparently supposed to perceive and appreciate that all the members were giving me unconditional love. I was supposed to learn to trust them, and I felt guilty if I couldn't. It was explained to me that I could not trust and believe that love existed at all because I hadn't received love in my dysfunctional family of origin. I took these explanations for granted because I was longing so much for love and wanted to believe that I actually was loved. I was unable to question what I was told, because hypocrisy had been the food I was fed daily by my mother – it was so familiar to me, though never questionable. But today I do question things that do not make sense to me.

Today I would say: Only a child needs (and absolutely needs) unconditional love. We must give it to the children who are entrusted to us. We must be able to love and accept them whatever they do, not only when they smile charmingly but also when they cry and scream. But to pretend to love an adult unconditionally – that is, independently of his or her deeds – would mean that we should love even a cold serial murderer or a notorious liar if only he joins our group. Can we do that? Should we even try? Why? For whose sake? If we say that we love an adult unconditionally, we only prove our blindness and/or dishonesty. Nothing else.

This is only one of many glimpses through the fog of religious heritage I tolerated in those meetings for much too long. I owe these insights to my lonely work. This ability to reason developed in me as I talked to my parents in my inner dialogue. It never occurred to me to have any conscious doubts when I was sitting in the meetings. I so desperately wanted to be loved – and that meant, of course, to comply, to be obedient. It was actually a very, very *conditional* 'love' that was being offered there.

Vera is right. As adults we don't need unconditional love, not even from our therapists. This is a childhood need, one that can never be fulfilled later in life, and we are playing with illusions if we have never mourned this lost opportunity. But there are other things we can get from good therapists: reliability, honesty, respect, trust, empathy, understanding, and an ability to clarify their emotions so that they need not bother us with them. If a therapist promises unconditional love, we must protect ourselves from him, from his hypocrisy and lack of awareness.

Vera was able to make an important discovery during her lonely work, thanks not only to the method she used but also to her determination to find the truth and not allow herself to be deceived again. The changes in her body, once she paid attention to it, supported her on her path.

Maja, thirty-eight, came to me several weeks after the birth of her third child and told me how free and alive she felt with this baby, quite in contrast to the way she had felt with her two previous children. With them she had constantly felt that excessive demands were being made upon her, that she was a prisoner, and that the babies were taking advantage of her and exploiting her. Thus she rebelled against their justified demands and, at the same time, felt that this was very bad of her: as in depression, she was separated from her true self. She thought these earlier reactions might actually have been rebellion against her mother's demands, for this time she was experiencing nothing of the sort. The love she had then struggled to feel now came of its own accord. She could enjoy her unity with this child and with herself. Then she spoke of her mother in the following words:

I was the jewel in my mother's crown. She often said: 'Maja can be relied upon, she will cope.' And I did cope. I brought up the smaller children for her so that she could get on with her professional career. She became more and more famous, but I never saw her happy. How often I longed for her in the evenings. The little ones cried and I comforted them but I myself never cried. Who would have wanted a crying child? I could only win my mother's love if I was competent, understanding, and controlled, if I never questioned her actions or showed her how much I missed her; that would have limited her freedom, which she needed so much. It would have turned her against me. At that time, nobody ever would have thought that this quiet, competent, useful Maja could be so lonely and have suffered so much. What could I do but be proud of my mother and help her? The deeper the hole in my mother's heart, the bigger the jewels in her crown needed to be. My poor mother needed these jewels because, at bottom, all her activity served only to suppress something in herself, perhaps a longing, I don't know. . . . Perhaps *she* would have discovered it if she had been fortunate enough to be a mother in more than a biological sense.

And how all of this repeated itself with Peter! How many empty hours my child had to spend with mother substitutes so that I could get my 'freedom,' which only took me further away from him and from myself. Now I know that I was looking for a way to avoid my feelings when I deserted him – without seeing what I was doing to him, because I had never been able to experience my own sense of being deserted. Only now do I begin to realize what motherhood without crown or jewels or a halo can be like.

A German women's magazine (which tries to speak openly of truths that have been taboo) published a reader's letter in which the tragic story of her experience of motherhood was told without disguise. Her report ends with the following passage:

And then the breast-feeding! The baby was put to the breast all wrong and soon my nipples were all bitten. God, how that hurt. Just two hours and then it was back: another one . . . the same. While it was sucking there, I was crying and swearing above it. It was so terrible that soon I couldn't eat any more and had a temperature of 40 degrees [Celsius]. Then I was allowed to wean and suddenly felt better. It was a long time before I noticed any maternal feelings. I wouldn't have minded if the baby had died. And everybody expected me to be happy. In despair I telephoned a friend who said that I'd get fond of him in time through being busy with him and having him around all the time. But that did not happen either. I only *began to be fond* of him when I could go back to work and only saw him when I came home, as a *distraction and toy*, so to speak. But quite honestly, a little dog would have done just as well. Now that he is gradually getting bigger and I see that I *can train him and that he is devoted to me and trusts me*, *I* am beginning to develop *tender feelings* for him and am glad that he is there.*

I have written all this because I think it is a good thing that someone should, at last, say that there is no such thing as mother love – not to speak of a maternal instinct. (*Emma*, July 1977)

This woman could not really experience either her own tragedy or that of her child, since her own emotionally inaccessible childhood was the real beginning

---

*Italics added.

and the actual key to this story. Her negative statement is thus incorrect. In truth, mother love and maternal instinct do exist; we can see them at work when we observe animals that have not been mistreated by human beings. Women, too, are born with instinctual programming to love, support, protect, and nurture their children and to derive pleasure from doing so. But we are robbed of these instinctual abilities if we are exploited in our childhood for the substitute gratification of our parents' needs. Fortunately, however, as Johanna's story shows, we can also restore these abilities as soon as we are determined to face our truth.

Johanna, age twenty-five, began her therapy just before she became pregnant. She was well prepared for the birth and enjoyed bonding with her healthy newborn. She was happy that her milk was abundant and was anticipating the joys of breast-feeding when suddenly, apparently without reason, her breasts became hard and painful and she developed a high fever. She was distraught when the nurse had to feed the baby with a bottle.

In her nightmares during the fever states, Johanna dreamed repeatedly and with many details of being sexually exploited in infancy by both of her parents and their friend. Thanks to the feelings that had been awakened in her self-therapy, she was able to feel her rage about the rape, the betrayal, and the damage to her instinctual capacity to fulfill her child's needs.

57

This last of her parents' crimes was what made her most furious. She said later: 'They robbed me of my maternal instincts when I was three months old. Because of what happened then, I was unable to breast-feed my child, although I wanted it so desperately.' It took a long time for her to confront her parents in an inner dialogue, to express all the feelings of rage and indignation that were stored up in her body, and finally to overcome the effects of these violations.

Even before this complete healing could take place, Johanna's willingness to face the horrible truth brought about a decrease in her temperature and an improvement in the condition of her breasts. She was able to feed her baby, who very quickly learned to dispense with the bottle. This came as a surprise to the nurse, who had been absolutely certain it 'would never work.'

Johanna was happy with her child. She enjoyed being able to love, to protect, to nurture, to hold her child, and to guess his needs. But this well-being was again and again interrupted by phases of doubt and fear that she would be confronted by catastrophic events if she continued to do what was simply a pleasure for her. As she had studied psychology, she wondered whether she suffered from an obsession and was just compelled to use her son for her own satisfaction, out of pure egoism. This painful self-condemnation was supported by her friends, who warned her about too much 'permissiveness' and instructed her that a child needs to learn his limits from the beginning. Otherwise he will become a tyrant. Although Johanna rejected these opinions for a long time, with her own child she was surprisingly sensitive to them and became quickly confused.

Therapy helped her to find orientation, again and again. And she found repeatedly how important it was to her just being able to love, to express her love without being afraid that she could be betrayed, exploited, violated. This love gave her the feeling of being whole, as she had been before her integrity had been injured. In her inner confrontation with her parents eventually, she said:

I love Michael, I want to love him. My soul needs this love like my body needs air. But I am so often in danger of suppressing my need with the help of my whole energy and my intellect. I think that I must 'free' myself from this attachment, that it is 'wrong.' Why? How have you brought me to feel these silly things? Maybe, by teaching me so early that a child doesn't deserve respect, that he is not a person, that he can be used as a toy to play with, that he can be ignored, mistreated, threatened without any consequences. It is this message, your message, that confuses me still from time to time, that makes me sometimes feel overdemanded and under stress, but I still do not dare to feel my rage toward you and become impatient with Michael. It seems easier to feel that it is Michael who hinders me to be free because he needs so much of my time. But it is not him. I only need to look at his eyes, to see his innocence and his honesty, and I know it: I have used him again as a scapegoat to protect you.

A loved child learns from the beginning what love is. A neglected, exploited, and mistreated child like me can't know it; she never had the chance to learn it. But I do learn it now, from Michael, very slowly, and I know that I will succeed, in spite of your messages. Because now I know how much I need to be able to love and no longer to have doubts about my ability.

I think that Johanna's struggle for her true feelings saved not only her child's future but also her own. Ann's story shows what can happen later to a molested child without this struggle, without therapy. Ann, fifty years old, wrote to me a few days before her death:

I had a visit from my adult children today and realized for the first time in my life that I have been loved by them, the whole time, and I never

Depression and Grandiosity

felt this love until today. I have abandoned them so often with various men and have actually been fleeing constantly from my children and my love for them, from my true feelings, into sexual pleasure with men who caused me so much pain and never gave me what I really needed: love, understanding, acceptance. As an infant I was conditioned by my father to look for pleasure connected with pain and rage and to avoid true love. Was it not a perversion? I was unable to escape it my whole life. And now, I can see it, but it is too late.

It was too late because, although Ann could see and understand what had happened to her, she was able to feel the rage and indignation only toward her partners, not toward her father. As she wrote in her letter, she still 'loved' and respected him.

DEPRESSIVE PHASES DURING THERAPY

A grandiose person will look for a therapist only if depressive episodes come to his aid and force him to do so. As long as the grandiose defense is effective, this form of disturbance exerts no pressure through visible suffering, except when other members of the family (spouse or children) have to seek psychotherapeutic help for depression or psychosomatic disorders. In

61

therapeutic work, we encounter grandiosity only when it is coupled with depression. On the other hand, we see depression in almost all our patients, either in the form of a manifest illness or in distinct phases of depressive moods. These phases can have different functions.

Signal Function

It happens quite often that a patient arrives complaining of depression and later leaves the consulting room in tears but much relieved and free from depression. Perhaps this patient has been able to experience a long-pent-up rage against her parent or has been able to express her mistrust. Perhaps she has felt for the first time her sadness over the many lost years of her life during which she did not really live, or has vented her anger over the impending holidays and separation from her therapist. It is irrelevant which of these feelings are coming to the fore; the important thing is that they can be experienced and that access is thereby allowed to repressed memories. The depression was a signal of both their proximity and their denial. A present event enabled the feelings to break through, and then the depression disappeared. Such a mood can be an indication that parts of the self that had been rejected (feelings, fantasies, wishes, fears) have become stronger, without being discharged in grandiosity.

Depression and Grandiosity

Suppression of Essential Needs

Mary, age thirty-nine, would sometimes leave a session feeling content and understood after having come close to the core of her self. But then she would distract herself with a party or something equally unimportant to her at that moment, which would make her feel lonely and inadequate again. After a few days she would complain of self-alienation and emptiness, of once more having lost the way to herself. In this way she was actively, though unconsciously, provoking a situation that could demonstrate what used to happen to her as a child: Whenever she began, through her imaginative play, to have a true sense of herself, her parents would ask her to do something 'more sensible' – to achieve something – and her inner world, which was just beginning to unfold, would be closed off to her. She reacted to this interference by withdrawing her feelings and becoming depressed, because she could not take the risk of a normal reaction – rage, perhaps.

If as an adult this person allows herself to face such reminders and work with them, she will be able to feel the old rage, rebel against the way she was treated, and find the repressed need. The depression will then disappear, because its defensive function is no longer needed. She will no longer have to flee into such activities as parties if she allows herself to know what she really needs at that very moment – possibly to *avoid* distraction and spend some time alone with herself in her plight.

The Accumulation of Strong, Hidden Feelings

Depressive phases may last several weeks before strong emotions from childhood break through. It is as though the depression has held back the affect. When it can be experienced, insight and associations related to the repressed scenes follow, often accompanied by significant dreams. The patient feels fully alive again until a new depressive phase signals something new. This may be expressed in the following fashion: 'I no longer have a feeling of myself. How could it happen that I should lose myself again? I have no connection with what is within me. It is all hopeless . . . it will never be any better. Everything is pointless. I am longing for my former sense of being alive.' An emotional outbreak may follow, accompanied by strong, legitimate reproaches, and only after this outbreak will a new link with repressed experience become clear and new vitality be felt. As long as these reproaches are directed toward those who are responsible for harming us, a great relief is the result. If, however, they are unjust, or transferred onto innocent persons, the depression will continue until full clarification becomes possible.

Depression and Grandiosity

Confronting the Parents

There will be times of depressive moods even after a person has started to resist the demands of his parents, as many things remain unconscious, repressed. He may, for example, resist their demands for achievement, although he has not yet fully freed himself from them. He will land again in the dead end of making pointlessly excessive demands upon himself and will become aware that he is doing so only when a depressive mood rises. He might, for example, report the following experience:

> The day before yesterday I was so happy. My work went easily – I was able to do more work for the exam than I had planned for the whole week. Then I thought I must take advantage of this good mood and do another chapter in the evening. I worked all evening but without any enthusiasm, and the next day I couldn't do any more. I felt like such an idiot. Nothing stayed in my head. I didn't want to see anyone, either; it felt like the depressions I used to have. Then I 'turned the pages back' and found the very moment it had begun. I had spoiled my pleasure as soon as I made myself do more and more. But why? Then I remembered how my mother used to say: 'You have done that beautifully, now you could surely do this too . . .'

I got very angry and left the books alone. Then, later, I trusted myself to know when I was ready to work again. And, of course, I did know. But the depression went away sooner – at the point when I got angry and realized how, and why, I had once again exceeded my limits.

THE INNER PRISON

Everyone probably knows about depressive moods from personal experience since they may be expressed as well as hidden by psychosomatic suffering. It is easy to notice, if we pay attention, that they hit almost with regularity – whenever we suppress an impulse or an unwanted emotion. Then, suddenly, a depressive mood will stifle all spontaneity. If an adult, for example, cannot experience grief when he loses somebody dear to him but tries to distract himself from his sadness, or if he suppresses* and hides from himself his indignation over an idealized friend's behavior out of fear of losing his friendship, he must reckon with the probability of depression (unless his grandiose defense is constantly at his disposal). When he begins to pay attention to these connections, he can benefit from his depression and use it to learn the truth about himself.

Once we have experienced a few times that the break-

*Suppression is a *conscious* act, in contrast to repression.

through of intense early-childhood feelings (character-ized by the specific quality of noncomprehension) can relieve a long period of depression, this experience will bring about a gradual change in our way of approaching 'undesired' feelings – painful feelings, above all. We dis-cover that we are no longer compelled to follow the former pattern of disappointment, suppression of pain, and depression, since we now have another possibility of dealing with disappointment: namely, experiencing the pain. In this way we at last gain access to our earlier experiences – to the parts of ourselves and our fate that were previously hidden from us.

A child does not yet have this possibility open to her. She cannot yet see through her mechanism of self-deception, and, on the other hand, she is far more threatened than an adult by the intensity of her feelings if she does not have a supportive, empathic environ-ment. Moreover, she can be in actual external danger. In contrast to the child, the adult is not in danger when she dares to feel, although she may, of course, fear the danger of her former situation (for the first time) as long as the reasons for her fear remain unconscious.

The extreme intensity of childhood feeling is to be found nowhere else, except in puberty. The recollec-tion of the pains of puberty, however – of not being able to understand or to place our own impulses – is usually more accessible than the earliest traumas, which are often hidden behind the picture of an idyllic childhood or even behind an almost complete amnesia. This is perhaps one reason why adults less often look back nostalgically to the time of their puberty than to that of their childhood. The mixture of longing, expectation, and fear of disappointment that for most people accompanies the remembrance of festivities from childhood can perhaps be explained by their search for the intensity of feeling they lost back then.

It is precisely because a child's feelings are so strong that they cannot be repressed without serious consequences. The stronger a prisoner is, the thicker the prison walls have to be, and unfortunately these walls also impede or completely prevent later emotional growth. In the closing phase of his therapy with me, a patient described the new understanding that came with the dismantling of his inner wall:

It was not the beautiful or pleasant feelings that gave me new insight, but the ones against which I had fought most strongly: feelings that made me experience myself as shabby, petty, mean, helpless, humiliated, demanding, resentful, or confused; and, above all, sad and lonely. It was precisely through these experiences, which I had shunned for so long, that I became certain that I now understand something about my life, stemming from the core of my being, something that I could not have learned from any book!

This patient was describing the process of gaining insight. Interpretations from therapists who ignore their own childhood history can disturb, hamper, and delay this process, or even prevent it or reduce it to mere intellectual insight. A person seeking help is all too ready to give up his own pleasure in discovery and self-expression and accommodate himself to his therapist's concepts, out of fear of losing the latter's affection, understanding, and empathy, for which he has been waiting all his life. Because of his early experiences with his mother, he cannot believe that this need not happen. If he gives way to this fear and adapts himself, the therapy slides over into the realm of the false self, and the true self remains hidden and undeveloped. It is therefore extremely important that the therapist not allow his own needs to impel him to formulate connections that the patient himself is discovering with the help of his own feelings. Otherwise he is in danger of behaving like a friend who brings a good meal to a prisoner in his cell, at the precise moment when that prisoner has the chance to escape – perhaps to spend his first night hungry and without shelter, but in freedom nevertheless. Since this first step into unknown territory would require a great deal of courage, the prisoner may comfort himself with his food and shelter and thus miss his chance and stay in prison.

Recognizing the fragility of the healing process obviously does not mean that the therapist must adopt a mostly silent and hurtful attitude, but merely that he must exercise care in this respect. It will then become possible for old, unremembered situations to be experienced consciously in their full tragedy for the first time and be mourned at last. Apparently, for many people that works more effectively without the help of therapists.

It is part of the dialectic of the grieving process that the experience of pain both encourages and is dependent on self-discovery. If the psychotherapist invites the patient to share in his own 'grandeur,' or if the patient is enabled to feel powerful as part of a therapeutic group, he will experience relief from his depression for a while, but the disturbance will still exist, appearing in a different guise for a time. Because grandiosity is the counterpart of depression *within* the narcissistic disturbance, the achievement of freedom from *both* forms of disturbance is hardly possible without deeply felt mourning about the situation of the former child. This ability to grieve – that is, to give up the illusion of his 'happy' childhood, to feel and recognize the full extent of the hurt he has endured – can restore the depressive's vitality and creativity and free the grandiose person from the exertions of and dependence on his Sisyphean task. If a person is able, during this long process, to experience the reality that he was never loved as a child for what he was but was instead needed and exploited for his achievements, success, and good qualities – and that he sacrificed his childhood for this form of love – he will be very deeply shaken, but one day he will feel the desire to end these efforts. He will discover in himself a need to live according to his true self and no longer be forced to earn 'love' that always leaves him empty-handed, since it is given to his false self – something he has begun to identify and relinquish.

The true opposite of depression is neither gaiety nor absence of pain, but vitality – the freedom to experience spontaneous feelings. It is part of the kaleidoscope of life that these feelings are not only happy, beautiful, or good but can reflect the entire range of human experience, including envy, jealousy, rage, disgust, greed, despair, and grief. But this freedom cannot be achieved if its childhood roots are cut off. Our access to the true self is possible only when we no longer have to be afraid of the intense emotional world of early childhood. Once we have experienced and become familiar with this world, it is no longer strange and threatening. We no longer need to keep it hidden behind the prison walls of illusion. We know now who and what caused our pain, and it is exactly this knowledge that gives us freedom at last from the old pain.

A good deal of advice for dealing with depression (for example, turning aggression from the inner to the outer world) has a clearly manipulative character. Some psychiatrists, for instance, suggest that the therapist should demonstrate to the patient that his hopelessness is not rational or make him aware of his oversensitivity. I think that such procedures will not only strengthen the false self and emotional conformity but will reinforce the depression as well. If therapists want to avoid doing so, they must take *all* of the patients' feelings seriously. How often depressive patients are aware that they have reacted oversensitively, and how much they reproach themselves for it. It is precisely their oversensitivity, shame, and self-reproach that form a continuous thread in their lives, unless they learn to understand to what these feelings actually relate. The more unrealistic such feelings are and the less they fit present reality, the more clearly they show that they are concerned with unremembered situations from the past that are still to be discovered. If the feeling that begins to arise is not experienced but reasoned away, the discovery cannot take place, and depression will triumph.

Pia, age forty, after a long depressive phase accompanied by suicidal thoughts, was at last able to experience and justify her long-suppressed rage toward her father, who had severely mistreated her. This experience was followed immediately not by visible relief, but by a period full of grief and tears. At the end of this period she said:

The world has not changed. There is so much evil

and meanness all around me, and I see it even more clearly than before. Nevertheless, for the first time I find life really worth living. Perhaps this is because, for the first time, I have the feeling that I am really living my own life. And that is an exciting adventure. On the other hand, I can understand my suicidal ideas better now, especially those I had in my youth – when it seemed pointless to carry on – because in a way I had always been living a life that wasn't mine, that I didn't want, and that I was ready to throw away.

A SOCIAL ASPECT OF DEPRESSION

One might ask whether adaptation must necessarily lead to depression. Is it not possible, and do we not sometimes see, that emotionally conforming individuals may live quite happily? There were perhaps many such examples in the past. Within a culture that was shielded from other value systems, an adapted individual was, of course, not autonomous. He did not have an individual sense of identity (in our sense) that could have given him support, but he felt supported by the group. Today it is hardly possible for any group to remain completely isolated from others with different values. The individual must therefore find his support within himself if he is to avoid becoming the victim of various interests and ideologies.

The so-called therapeutic groups try to but cannot provide or replace this maturational process. Their goal is to 'empower' their members by providing them with support and a sense of belonging. Since the suppression of childhood feelings is the rule within these groups, however, the individual's depression cannot be resolved. Moreover, a person can become addicted to the group itself, as the group provides the *illusion* that the unmet needs of the former child can eventually be fulfilled (by the group) in the adult. With such illusions, no one can truly heal. The strength within ourselves – through access to our own real needs and feelings and the possibility of expressing them – is crucially important for us if we want to live without depression and addiction.

Some children have latent powers to resist adaptation and become partially adapted. Older children, particularly as they reach puberty, may attach themselves to new values, which are often opposed to those of the parents. An adolescent may accept and conform to the ideals of a group of youths just as he did to those of his parents when he was younger. But since this attempt is not rooted in an awareness of his own true needs and feelings, he is again giving up and denying his true self in order to be accepted and loved, this time by a peer group. His renewed sacrifice will therefore not relieve his depression. He is not really himself, nor does he know or love himself: Everything he undertakes is done in hope of making somebody love him in the way he once, as a child, so urgently needed to be loved; but what could not be experienced at the appropriate time in the past can never be attained later on.

There are innumerable examples of this dilemma. I will describe two of them:

1: Paula, age twenty-eight, wanted to free herself from her patriarchal family in which the mother was completely subjugated by the father. She married a submissive man and seemed to behave differently from her mother. Her husband allowed her to bring her lovers into the house. She did not permit herself any feelings of jealousy or tenderness and wanted to have relations with a number of men without any emotional ties, so that she could feel as autonomous as a man. Her need to be 'progressive' went so far that she allowed her partners to abuse and humiliate her, and she suppressed all her feelings of mortification and anger in the belief that her behavior made her modern and free from prejudice. In this way she unconsciously carried over into these relationships both her childhood obedience and her mother's submissiveness. At times she suffered from severe depression, so she entered therapy, which enabled her to feel how much she suffered because of the passiveness of her mother, who tolerated the abusive father without the slightest opposition. Confronting the pain of not having been protected by her indifferent, defensive mother eventually helped Paula to stop creating her mother's self-destructive attitude in her own relationships with men and to allow herself to love people who deserved her love.

2: Amar, now forty, grew up in an African family, alone with his mother after his father died when he was still a very small boy. His mother insisted on certain conventions and did not allow him to be aware of his needs in any way, let alone express them. On the other hand, she regularly massaged his penis until puberty, ostensibly on medical advice. As an adult, the son left his mother and her world and married an attractive European with a different background. Due to his repressed history, he chose a woman who not only tormented and humiliated him but also undermined his confidence to an extreme degree, so that he was unable either to stand up to her or to leave her.

This sadomasochistic marriage, like the other example, represents an attempt to break away from the parents' social system with the help of another one. Amar was certainly able to free himself from the mother of his adolescence, but he remained emotionally tied to the mother of his early childhood (and his unconscious memories of her), whose role was taken over by his wife as long as he was not able to experience the feelings from that period. It was terribly painful for him to realize how much he had needed his mother as a child and at the same time had felt abused in his helplessness – how much he had loved her, hated her, and been entirely at her mercy. But as a result of this experience, Amar no longer feared his wife and for the first time dared to see her as she really was.

The child must adapt to ensure the illusion of love, care, and kindness, but the adult does not need this illusion to survive. He can give up his amnesia and then be in a position to determine his actions with open eyes. Only this path will free him from his depression. Both the depressive and the grandiose person *completely deny their childhood reality* by living as though the availability of the parents could still be salvaged: the grandiose person through the illusion of achievement, and the depressive through his constant fear of losing 'love.' Neither can accept the truth that this loss or absence of love has *already happened* in the past, and that *no effort whatsoever can change this fact.*

THE LEGEND OF NARCISSUS

The legend of Narcissus actually tells us the tragedy of the loss of the self. Narcissus sees his reflection in the water and falls in love with his own beautiful face, of which his mother was surely proud. The nymph Echo answers the young man's calls because she is in love with his beauty. Echo's answering calls deceive Narcissus. His reflection deceives him as well, since it shows only his perfect, wonderful face and not his inner world, his pain, his history. His back view, for instance, and his shadow remain hidden from him; they do not belong to and are cut off from his beloved reflection.

This stage of rapturous enchantment can be compared to grandiosity, just as the next (the consuming longing for himself) can be likened to depression. Narcissus wanted to be nothing but the beautiful youth; he totally denied his true self. In trying to be at one with the beautiful picture, he gave himself up – to death or, in Ovid's version, to being changed into a flower. This death is the logical consequence of the fixation on the false self. It is not only the 'beautiful,' 'good,' and pleasant feelings that make us really alive, deepen our existence, and give us crucial insight, but often precisely the unacceptable and unadapted ones from which we would prefer to escape: helplessness, shame, envy, jealousy, confusion, rage, and grief. These feelings can be experienced in therapy. When they are understood, they open the door to our inner world that is much richer than the 'beautiful countenance'!

Narcissus was in love with his idealized picture, but neither the grandiose nor the depressive 'Narcissus' can really love himself. His passion for his false self makes impossible not only love for others but also, despite all appearances, love for the one person who is fully entrusted to his care: himself.

3

The Vicious Circle of Contempt

Would not God find a way out, some superior deception such as the grownups and the powerful always contrived, producing one more trump card at the last moment, shaming me after all, not taking me seriously, humiliating me under the damnable mask of kindness?

HERMANN HESSE, 'A CHILD'S HEART'

HUMILIATION FOR THE CHILD, DISRESPECT FOR THE WEAK, AND WHERE IT GOES FROM THERE

While away on a vacation, I was sorting out my thoughts on the subject of contempt and reading various notes I had made on this theme after individual sessions. Probably sensitized by this preoccupation, I was more than usually affected by an ordinary scene, in no way spectacular or rare. I shall describe it to introduce my observations, for it illustrates, without any danger of indiscretion, some of the insights I have gained in my work.

I was out for a walk and noticed a young couple a few steps ahead, both tall; they had a little boy with them, about two years old, who was running alongside and whining. (We are accustomed to seeing such situations from the adult point of view, but here I want to describe it as experienced by the child.) The two had just bought themselves ice-cream bars on sticks from the kiosk, and were licking them with evident enjoyment. The little boy wanted one, too His mother said affectionately, 'Look, you can have a bite of mine, a whole one is too cold for you.' The child did not want just one bite but held out his hand for the whole bar, which his mother took out of his reach again. He cried in despair, and soon exactly the same thing was repeated with his father: 'There you are, my pet,' said his father affectionately, 'you can have a bite of mine.' 'No, no,' cried the child and ran ahead again, trying to distract himself. Soon he came back again and gazed enviously and sadly up at the two grown-ups, who were enjoying their ice cream contentedly. Time and again he held out his little hand for the whole ice-cream bar, but the adult hand with its treasure was withdrawn again.

The more the child cried, the more it amused his parents. It made them laugh, and they hoped to humor him along with their laughter, too: 'Look, it isn't so important, what a fuss you are making.' Once the child sat down on the ground and began to throw little stones over his shoulder in his mother's direction, but then he suddenly got up again and looked around anxiously, making sure that his parents were still there. When his father had completely finished his ice cream, he gave the stick to the child and walked on. The little boy licked the bit of wood expectantly, looked at it, threw it away, wanted to pick it up again but did not do so, and a deep sob of loneliness and disappointment shook his small body. Then he trotted obediently after his parents.

It seemed clear to me that this little boy was not being frustrated in his 'oral wishes,' for he was given ample opportunity to take a bite; he was, however, constantly being hurt and frustrated. His wish to hold the ice-cream stick in his hand like the others was not understood. Worse still, it was laughed at; they made fun of his wish. He was faced with two giants who supported each other and who were proud of being consistent while he, quite alone in his distress, could say nothing beyond 'no.' Nor could he make himself clear to his parents with his gestures (though they were very expressive). He had no advocate. What an unfair situation it is when a child is opposed by two big, strong adults, as by a wall; but we call it 'consistency in upbringing' when we refuse to let the child complain about one parent to the other.

Why, indeed, did these parents behave with so little empathy? Why didn't one of them think of eating a little quicker, or even of throwing away half of the ice cream and giving the child the stick with a bit of ice cream left on it? Why did they both stand there laughing, eating so slowly and showing so little concern about the child's obvious distress? They were not unkind or cold parents; the father spoke to his child very tenderly. Nevertheless, at least at this moment, they displayed a lack of empathy.

We can only solve this riddle if we manage to see the parents, too, as insecure children – children who have at last found a weaker creature, in comparison with whom they can now feel very strong. What child has never been laughed at for his fears and been told, 'You don't need to be afraid of a thing like that'? What child will then not feel shamed and despised because he could not assess the danger correctly? And will that little person not take the next opportunity to pass these feelings on to a still smaller child? Such experiences come in all shades and varieties. Common to them all is the sense of strength it gives the adult, who cannot control his or her own fears, to face the weak and helpless child's fear and be able to control fear in another person.

No doubt, in twenty years' time – or perhaps earlier if he has younger siblings – our little boy will replay this scene with the ice cream. Now, however, *he* will be in charge, and the other will be the helpless, envious, weak little creature – no longer carried within, but split off and projected outside himself.

Disregard for those who are smaller and weaker is thus the best defense against a breakthrough of one's own feelings of helplessness: it is an expression of this split-off weakness. The strong person who – because he has experienced it – knows that he, too, carries this weakness within himself does not need to demonstrate his strength through contempt.

Many adults first become aware of their feelings of helplessness, jealousy, and loneliness through their own children, since they had no chance to acknowledge and experience these feelings consciously in childhood. I've spoken of the patient Peter who was obsessively forced to make conquests with women, to seduce and then to abandon them, until he was at last able to experience how he himself had repeatedly been abandoned by his mother (p. 20). When he also remembered how he had been laughed at by his parents, he consciously experienced for the first time the feelings of humiliation and mortification that were aroused back then. Until that point, all of these feelings had been completely concealed from his consciousness.

The suffering that was not consciously felt as a child can be avoided by delegating it to one's own children – in much the same way as in the ice-cream scene I have just described: 'You see, we are big, we may do as we like, but for you it is "too cold." You may enjoy yourself as we do only when you get to be big enough.' So it is not the frustration of his wish that is humiliating for the child, but the contempt shown for his person. The suffering is accentuated by the parents' demonstrating their 'grown-upness' to avenge themselves unconsciously on their child for their own earlier humiliation. They encounter their own humiliating past in the child's eyes, and they ward it off with the power they now have. We cannot, simply by an act of will, free ourselves from repeating the patterns of our parents' behavior – which we had to learn very early in life. We become free of them only when we can fully feel and acknowledge the suffering they inflicted on us. We can then become fully aware of these patterns and condemn them unequivocally.

In most societies, little girls suffer additional discrimination because they are girls. Since women, however, usually have control of newborn infants and toddlers, these former little girls can pass on to their children at the most tender age the disrespect from which they once suffered. When that happens, the grown son will idealize his mother, since every human being needs the feeling (and clings to the illusion) that he was really loved; but he will despise other women, upon whom he can take revenge in place of his mother. And the humiliated grown daughter, if she has no other means of ridding herself of her burden, will revenge herself upon her own children. She can do so secretly and without fear of reprisals, for the children have no way of telling anyone, except perhaps later in the form of obsessions or other symptoms, the language of which is sufficiently veiled that the mother is not betrayed.

Disrespect is the weapon of the weak and a defense against one's own despised and unwanted feelings, which could trigger memories of events in one's repressed history. And the fountainhead of all contempt, all discrimination, is the more or less conscious, uncontrolled, and covert exercise of power over the child by the adult. Except in the case of murder or serious bodily harm, this unrestrained use of power is tolerated by society; what adults do to their child's spirit is entirely their own affair, for the child is regarded as the parents' property in the same way as the citizens of a totalitarian state are considered the property of its government. Until we become sensitized to the small child's suffering, this wielding of power by adults will continue to be regarded as a normal aspect of the human condition, for hardly anyone pays attention to it or takes it seriously. Because the victims are 'only children,' their distress is trivialized. But in twenty years' time these children will be adults who will feel compelled to pay it all back to their own children. They may consciously fight with vigor against cruelty in the world yet carry within themselves an experience of cruelty that they may unconsciously inflict on others. As long as it remains hidden behind their idealized picture of a happy childhood, they will have no awareness of it and will therefore be unable to avoid passing it on.

It is absolutely urgent that people become aware of the degree to which this disrespect of children is persistently transmitted from one generation to the next, perpetuating destructive behavior. Someone who slaps or hits another adult or knowingly insults her is aware of hurting her. Even if he doesn't know why he is doing this, he has some sense of what he is doing. But how often were our parents, and we ourselves toward our own children, unconscious of how painfully, deeply, and abidingly they and we injured a child's tender, budding self?

It is very fortunate when our older children become aware of what we were doing and are able to tell us about it. We are then given the opportunity to recognize our failures and to apologize. Acknowledging what we have done may help them, at last, to throw off the chains of neglect, discrimination, scorn, and misuse of power that have been handed on for generations. When our children can consciously experience their early helplessness and rage, they will no longer need to ward off these feelings, in turn, with the exercise of power over others. In most cases, however, people's childhood suffering remains affectively inaccessible and thus forms the hidden source of new and sometimes very subtle humiliation for the next generation. Various defense mechanisms will help to justify their actions: denial of their own suffering, rationalization (I owe it to my child to bring him up properly), displacement (it is not my father but my son who is hurting me), idealization (my father's beatings were good for me), and more. Above all, there is the mechanism of turning repressed suffering into active behavior. The following examples may illustrate how astonishingly similar the ways are in which people protect themselves against their childhood experiences, despite great differences in personality structure and education.

A thirty-year-old Greek, the son of a peasant and owner of a small restaurant in Western Europe, proudly described how he drinks no alcohol and has his father to thank for this abstinence. Once, at the age of fifteen, he came home drunk and was so severely beaten by his father that he could not move for a week. From that time on he was so averse to alcohol that he could not taste so much as a drop, although his work brought him into constant contact with it. When I heard that he was soon to be married, I asked whether he, too, would beat his children. 'Of course,' he answered. 'Beatings are necessary in bringing up a child properly. They are the best way to make him respect you. I would never smoke in my father's presence, for example – and that is a sign of my respect for him.'

This man was neither stupid nor coldhearted, but he

had received little schooling. We might therefore nurse the illusion that education could counteract this on-going process of destroying the spirit. But how does this idea stand up to the next example, which concerns an educated man?

In the seventies, a talented Czech author was reading from his own works in a town in Western Germany. After the reading there followed a discussion with the audience, during which he was asked questions about his life. He answered ingenuously, reporting that despite his former support of the Prague Spring he now had plenty of freedom and could travel frequently in the West. He went on to describe his country's development in recent years. When he was asked about his childhood, his eyes shone with enthusiasm as he talked about his gifted and many-sided father, who encouraged his spiritual development and was a true friend. It was only to his father that he could show his first stories. His father was very proud of him, and even when he beat him as punishment for some misdemeanor reported by the mother, he was proud that his son did not cry. Since tears brought extra blows, the child learned to suppress them and was himself proud that he could make his admired father such a great present with his bravery. This man spoke of these regular beatings as though they were the most normal things in the world (as for him, of course, they were), and then he said: 'It did me no harm, it prepared me for life, made me hard, taught me to grit my teeth. And that's why I could get on so well in my profession.' And it was also for that reason that he could cooperate so well with the Communist totalitarian regime.

In contrast with this Czech author, the film director Ingmar Bergman spoke on a television program with more understanding and greater – although only intellectual – awareness about the implications of his own childhood, which he described as one long story of humiliation. He related, for example, that if he wet his pants he had to wear a red dress all day so that everybody would know what he had done and he would be ashamed of himself. Bergman, the younger son of a Protestant pastor, described in this television interview a scene that often occurred during his childhood: His older brother has just been beaten by the father. Now their mother is dabbing his brother's bleeding back with cotton, while he himself sits watching. The adult Bergman described this scene without apparent agitation, coldly. One could see him as a child, quietly sitting and watching. He surely did not run away, or close his eyes, or cry. One had the impression that this scene did take place in reality but was at the same time a covering memory for what *he himself* went through. It is unlikely that only his brother was beaten by their father.

Sometimes people are convinced that it was just their

siblings who suffered humiliation. Only in therapy can they remember – with feelings of rage and helplessness, of anger and indignation – how humiliated and deserted they felt when they themselves were mercilessly beaten by their beloved father.

Ingmar Bergman, however, had another means, apart from projection and denial, of dealing with his suffering: He could make films and thereby delegate his unfelt feelings to the spectator. We, as the movie audience, are asked to endure those feelings that he, the son of such a father, could not experience overtly but nevertheless carried within himself. We sit before the screen confronted, the way that small boy once was, with all the cruelty 'our brother' has to endure, and feel hardly able or willing to take in all this brutality with authentic feelings; we ward them off.

Bergman also spoke regretfully of his failure to see through Nazism before 1945, although as an adolescent he often visited Germany during the Hitler period. I see this blindness as a consequence of his childhood. Cruelty was the familiar air he had breathed from early on, so why should cruelty and disdain for others have caught his attention?

And why have I described three examples of men who were beaten in their childhood? Are these not borderline cases? Do I want to consider only the effects of beatings? By no means. I chose these three cases, although they *may* be crass exceptions, partly because they had not been entrusted to me as secrets but had already been made public; but above all, I meant to show how the impact of even the most severe ill-treatment can remain hidden because of the child's strong tendency to idealization. There is no trail, no advocate, no verdict. Everything remains shrouded in the darkness of the past; and should the facts become known, they appear in the guise of 'blessings.' If this is so with the most blatant examples of physical mistreatment, then how is emotional torment ever to be exposed, when it is less visible and more easily disputed? Who is likely to take serious notice of subtle discrimination, as in the example of the small boy and the ice cream? But each patient's therapy reveals endless comparable examples.

The parent's exploitation of their child can lead to a long series of sexual and nonsexual abuses, which the child will be able to discover only as an adult in therapy, and often not before he himself is a parent. A father who grew up in a puritanical family may well be inhibited in his sexual relationships in marriage. He may even first dare to look closely at female genitalia, play with them, and feel aroused while he is bathing his small daughter. A mother may perhaps have been shocked as a small girl by the unexpected sight of an erect penis and so developed fear of the male genital, or she may have experienced it as an implement of violence without being able to confide in anyone. Such a mother may now be able to feel she has gained control over her fear in relationship to her tiny son. She may, for example, dry him after his bath in such a manner that he has an erection, which is not dangerous or threatening for her. She may massage her son's penis, right up to puberty, in order 'to treat a constriction of his foreskin' without having to be afraid. Protected by the unquestioning love that every child has for his mother, she can carry on with her hesitant sexual exploration, which never had a chance to develop naturally.

What does it mean to the child, however, when her inhibited parents exploit her sexually? Every child seeks loving contact and is happy to get it, but at the same time feels confused, insecure, and afraid when a mixture of feelings is elicited that would not appear spontaneously at this stage in her development. Her fear and confusion are further increased when her own autoerotic activity is punished by the parents' prohibitions or scorn.

There are other ways of exploiting the child apart from the sexual: through brainwashing, for instance, which underlies both the 'anti-authoritarian' and the 'strict' upbringing. Neither form of rearing takes the child's own needs into account. As soon as he is regarded as a *possession* for which one has a particular *goal,* as soon as one exerts control over him, his natural growth will be violently interrupted.

It is among the commonplaces of education that we often first cut off the living root and then try to replace its natural functions by artificial means. Thus we suppress the child's curiosity, for example (there are questions one should not ask), and then when he lacks a natural interest in learning we offer him special coaching for his scholastic difficulties.

We find a similar example in the behavior of addicts. People who as children successfully repressed their intense feelings often try to regain – at least for a short time – their lost intensity of experience with the help of drugs or alcohol. (See Miller 1983, pp. 107–141.)

If we want to avoid unconsciously motivated exploitation and disrespect of the child, we must first gain a conscious awareness of these dangers. Only if we become sensitive to the fine and subtle ways (as well as the more obvious but still denied ways) in which a child may suffer humiliation can we hope to develop the respect for him he will need from the very first day of his life. There are various means of developing this sensitivity. We may, for instance, observe children who are strangers to us and attempt to feel empathy for them in their situation. But we must, above all, come to have empathy for our own fate. Our feelings will always reveal the true story, which no one else knows and which only we can discover.

WORKING WITH CONTEMPT IN THERAPY

When I worked as a psychoanalyst I was sometimes asked in seminars or supervisors' sessions how one should deal with 'undesirable' feelings such as the irritation that patients sometimes arouse in the therapist. A sensitive therapist will of course feel this irritation. Should he suppress it in order to avoid rejecting the patient? But then the patient, too, will sense this suppressed anger, without being able to comprehend it, and will be confused. Should the therapist express it? Doing so may offend the patient and undermine her confidence. The question of how to deal with anger and other unwanted feelings toward the patient no longer needs to be asked if we begin with the assumption that *all* the feelings the patient arouses in her therapist or counselor are part of her unconscious attempt to tell the therapist her story and at the same time to hide it from him. Although the way a patient evokes fear or irritation in the therapist is of course due in part to the patient's history, these feelings can also, in large part, be triggered by the therapist's own past. They should not be warded off, for they always indicate a hidden reality and past knowledge. The therapist must be able to experience them and clear them up. He must find out whether the feelings provoked by the patient are being triggered by his own life history; and if so, he will be able to work on them. The same relates to counselors who work with addicted patients or other victims of sexual or physical childhood mistreatment. Usually, they sense only a trace of their own fear before quickly concealing it with the help of abstract theories, commonplace moral advice, or very often simply authoritarian behavior.

Damaged Self-Articulation in the Compulsion to Repeat

The newly won capacity to accept her feelings opens the way for the patient's long-repressed needs and wishes to be actualized. Some of these needs cannot be satisfied in reality, since they are related to past situations. The urgent wish for a child, for example, may express among other things the wish to have an available mother. Unfortunately, children are too often wished for only as symbols to meet repressed needs.

All the same, there are needs that can and should be satisfied in the present. Among these is every human being's central need to express herself, to show herself to the world as she really is – in word, in gesture, in behavior, in art – in every genuine expression, beginning with the baby's cry.

For the person who, as a child, had to hide her true feelings from herself and others, this first step into the open produces much anxiety, yet she feels a great need to throw over her former restraints. The first experiences do not always lead to freedom but quite often lead instead to a repetition of the person's childhood situation, in which she will experience feelings of agonizing shame and painful nakedness as an accompaniment to her genuine expressions of her true self. With the infallibility of a sleepwalker, she will seek out those who, like her parents (though for different reasons), certainly cannot understand her. Because of her blindness caused by repression, she will try to make herself understandable to precisely these people – trying to make possible what cannot be.

During her therapy, Linda, forty-two, fell in love with an older, intelligent, and sensitive man, who nevertheless had to ward off and reject everything – except for eroticism – he could not understand intellectually, including psychotherapy. Yet he was the one to whom she wrote long letters trying to explain the path she had taken in her therapy up to this point. She succeeded in overlooking all signals of his incomprehension and increased her efforts even more, until at last she was forced to recognize that she had again found a father substitute and that this was the reason she had been unable to give up her hopes of at last being understood. This awakening brought her agonizingly sharp feelings of shame, which lasted for a long time.

One day she was able to feel this shame deeply in the session and said: 'I feel so ridiculous, as if I've been talking to a wall and expecting it to answer, like a silly child.' I asked: 'Would you think it ridiculous if you saw a child who had to tell his troubles to a wall because there was no one else available?' The despairing sobbing that followed my question gave Linda access to a part of her former reality that was pervaded by boundless loneliness. It also eventually freed her from her agonizing, self-destructive, repetitive feelings of shame.

Only much later could Linda dare to connect this experience of 'a wall' with her own childhood history. For a time this woman, who was normally capable of expressing herself so clearly, described everything in such an extraordinarily complicated way and at such precipitate speed that I couldn't fully understand it. She went through moments of sudden hate and rage, reproaching me for indifference and lack of understanding. Linda could hardly recognize me anymore, although I had not changed. In her estranged feelings she now discovered the estrangement of her mother, who had spent the first year of her life in an orphanage and could not give her daughter any tenderness or closeness. Linda had known that for a long time, but it was only intellectual knowledge. Moreover, compassion for her mother's sad life history had hindered Linda from feeling her own plight; the image of the poor mother had blocked her feelings.

It was not until she could make her reproaches, first

toward me and then toward her mother, that the core of her despair became conscious: her lifelong search for closeness and contact that had never been met in infancy and had become repressed. Repressed memories of the shy, distant, absent mother produced in the daughter the feeling of a wall, one that later separated her from other people in such a painful way. She was finally released from a compulsion to repeat that had consisted of constantly seeking a partner who had no understanding of her and then allowing herself to settle into an arrangement where she would feel helplessly dependent on him. The fascination of such tormenting relationships is a result of repressed memories and the struggle for a better outlet at last.

Perpetuation of Contempt in Perversion and Obsessive Behavior

If we start from the premise that a person's whole development (and his balance, which is based upon it) is dependent on the way *his mother* experienced his *expression of needs and sensations* during his first days and weeks of life, then we must assume that it is here that the *beginning of a later tragedy* might be set. If a mother cannot take pleasure in her child as he is but must have him behave in a particular way, then the first value selection takes place for the child. Now 'good' is differentiated from 'bad,' 'nice' from 'nasty,' and 'right' from 'wrong.' Against this background will follow all his further valuations of himself.

Such an infant must learn that there are things about him for which the mother has 'no use.' She will expect her child to control his bodily functions as early as possible. On the conscious level his parents apparently want him to do so in order not to offend against society, but unconsciously they are protecting their own repression dating from the time when they were themselves small children afraid of 'offending.'

Marie Hesse, the mother of the poet and novelist Hermann Hesse, described in her diaries how her own will was broken at the age of four. When her son was four years old, she suffered greatly under his defiant behavior and battled against it with varying degrees of success. At the age of fifteen, Hermann Hesse was sent to an institution for the care of epileptics and defectives in Stetten, 'to put an end to his defiance once and for all.' In an affecting and angry letter from Stetten, Hesse wrote to his parents: 'If I were a bigot, and not a human being, I could perhaps hope for your understanding.' All the same, his release from the home was made conditional upon his 'improvement,' and so the boy 'improved.'

In a later poem dedicated to his parents, denial and idealization are restored: he reproaches *himself* that it had been 'his character' that had made life so difficult for his parents. Many people suffer all their lives from this oppressive feeling of guilt, the sense of not having lived up to their parents' expectations. This feeling is stronger than any intellectual insight they might have, that it is not a child's task or duty to satisfy his parent's needs. No argument can overcome these guilt feelings, for they have their beginnings in life's earliest period, and from that they derive their intensity and obduracy. They can be resolved only slowly, with the help of a revealing therapy.

Probably the greatest of wounds – not to have been loved just as one truly was – cannot heal without the work of mourning. It can be either more or less successfully resisted and covered up (as in grandiosity and depression), or constantly torn open again in the compulsion to repeat. We encounter this latter possibility in obsessive behavior and in perversion, where the mother's (or father's) scornful reactions to the child's behavior have stayed with him as repressed memory, stored up in his body. (The same happens with mistreatments and molestations that have been endured.) The mother often reacted with surprise and horror, aversion and disgust, shock and indignation, or fear and panic to the child's most natural impulses – his autoerotic behavior, investigation and discovery of his own body, urination and defecation, or his curiosity or rage in response to betrayal and injustice. Later, all these experiences remain closely linked with the mother's horrified eyes. They drive the former child to obsessions and perversions in which the traumatic scenes that were endured can be reproduced. In order for pain to be avoided, the true meaning of these scenes must remain unrecognizable to the person himself.

The patient goes through torment when he reveals to the therapist his hitherto secret sexual and auto-erotic behavior. He may, of course, also relate this material quite unemotionally, merely giving information, as if speaking of some other person. Such a report, however, will neither help him break out of his loneliness nor lead him back to the reality of his childhood. It is only when he is willing not to fend off his feelings of shame and fear, but rather to accept and experience them, that he can discover the real past reasons for these feelings. His most harmless behavior will then cause him to feel mean, dirty, or completely annihilated. He is surprised indeed when he realizes how long this repressed feeling of shame has survived, and how it has found a place alongside his tolerant and advanced views of sexuality. These experiences first show the person that his early adaptation by means of splitting was not an expression of cowardice, but that it was really his only chance to survive, to escape his fear of annihilation.

Can a mother be so menacing? Yes, if she was always proud of being her mother's dear, good daughter, who was dry at the age of six months and clean at a year, who at three could 'mother' her younger siblings, and so forth.* In her own baby, such a mother sees the split-off and never-experienced part of her self, of whose breakthrough into consciousness she is afraid. She also sees the uninhibited sibling baby, whom she mothered at such an early age and only now envies and perhaps hates in the person of her own child. So she trains her child with looks, despite what may be a greater intellectual wisdom than her own mother's.

As the child grows up, he cannot cease living his own truth and expressing it somewhere, perhaps in complete secrecy. In this way a person can have adapted completely to the demands of his surroundings and can have developed a false self, but in his perversion of his obsessions he still allows a portion of his true self to survive – in torment. And so the true self lives on, but underground, in the same conditions as the child once did with his disgusted mother, whose memory in the meantime he has repressed. In his perversion and obsessions he constantly reenacts the same drama: A horrified mother is necessary before sexual satisfaction is possible; orgasm (for instance, with a fetish) can be achieved only in a climate of self-

*This particular form of tampering with a child's natural development may not be as familiar to readers in the United States as it is in Europe. Many of my patients were dry at five months, and their mothers were quite proud of this 'achievement.' American readers may be better acquainted with such practices as scheduled feedings and training infants to sleep through the night by ignoring their cries.

contempt; criticism can be expressed only in (seem-ingly) absurd, unaccountable, and frightening obsessive fantasies. Nothing will better serve to acquaint us with the hidden tragedy of certain uncon-scious mother-child relationships than witnessing the destructive power of the compulsion to repeat, and that compulsion's dumb, unconscious communica-tion in the shaping of its drama.

It is of primary importance that, although the patient may *experience* the therapist as hostile to his desires and compulsions, critical and contemptuous, the therapist should never in fact really be so. This may sound obvi-ous, but it is not always true in practice. In fact, the therapist sometimes does just the opposite, quite unconsciously. Because he fears his own repressed terror, he may be unable to bear being turned into a hostile figure and may demonstrate his tolerance in a way that does not allow the child's fear and confusion to come up in the patient.

Such a therapist may emphasize that his patients are for him *always* adult clients and not 'children' – as if the feelings of a child were something to be ashamed of, and not something valuable and helpful. Occasionally one hears similar remarks about sickness, when a ther-apist is eager to consider his patients as healthy as possible; he may warn them against 'dangerous regres-sion,' as if 'sickness' were not sometimes the only possible way of expressing the person's plight. Many people have, after all, been trying all their lives to be as adult and healthy (normal) as possible. They should be given support for the relief they feel at the discovery of this socially conditioned straitjacket of child-rejection and 'normalcy-worship' within themselves. By giving it up they will get in touch with their true feelings. This is one of the reasons I prefer to use the word 'patient' instead of 'client,' which is more frequently used by therapists today. It was not until I experienced myself as a patient, as a suffering person, that I could find my way out of the trap of repression and help myself. As the 'client' of (seemingly) 'good therapists,' I could find only *their* knowledge, something which was of no help at all in my quest for healing.

Mark, thirty-two, who suffered under his perversion and constantly feared the rejection of others, bore within himself the unconscious memory of his mother's rejection. Without knowing why, he was compelled to do things that his social circle and society in general disapprove of and despise, although he feared the punishment he was provoking. If society were suddenly to have honored his form of perversion (as happens in certain circles), he would perhaps have had to change his compulsion, but that would never have freed him. What he was compelled to seek was not permission to use one or another fetish, but – with the hope for a better outcome – his mother's disgusted and horrified eyes. He looked for this response in his therapist, too, using all possible means to provoke him to disgust, horror, and aversion. This provocation of course recounted what had actually happened at the beginning of Mark's life. This recounting was of no use to him, however, as long as the old feelings were blocked. The most brilliant intellect cannot break this block down. But with the help of his complaints, the experience of profound feelings, with confronting the abuses and condemning the deeds – he could give up his acting out. He now knew what he *really* needed.

If a person can see through to the goals and compulsions behind this sort of provocation, then the whole decayed building collapses and gives way to true, deep, and defenseless mourning. When this happens, all the distortions are no longer necessary. This is a clear demonstration of how mistaken the attempt is to show a patient his 'sexual conflicts' if he has been trained from earliest childhood on to *feel nothing*. How can these conflicts be experienced without feelings of rage, abandonment, jealousy, loneliness, love?

In the last ten years I have received many letters from readers who wrote to me to say that as teenagers they had been sexually abused, seduced, and emotionally exploited by adult men, without ever being able to recognize this fact because of their blindness stemming from repressed childhood memories. It was not before they read my book *Thou Shalt Not Be Aware* that they began to have doubts and suspicions. For the first time in their lives, they dared to question the behavior of their perpetrators. The idea that they had been betrayed, that their longing for love and affection had been exploited, never before occurred to them, because they were unable to feel. The only path available to them was to idealize the seducer, the big friend, savior, teacher, master, and to become addicted to a special form of sexual behavior, or to drugs, or to both. Struggling for social acceptance of special forms of addictions, sexual and nonsexual, is one of the many ways to avoid confrontation with our own history.

There are many people whose needs for protection, care, and tenderness, whose unmet longing for love, were very early sexualized and who lived their lives with various sexual fixations without ever having faced their history. They join groups, accept uncritically theories that confirm their fixations, and pretend to share with others 'scientific' knowledge, while they unconsciously disguise their own repressed history. As long as they do, they damage others in the same way they have been damaged, without any remorse.

I think that the future (the therapy) of these people and their victims is jeopardized by every kind of ideology. They should rather be informed that it is possible to discover one's history, to work it through, and to liberate oneself from fixations that can be destructive for oneself and others. It is very striking to see how often a sexual 'addiction' ceases when the patient begins to experience *his own* feelings and can recognize his *true* needs.

The following quote is taken from a report about St. Pauli, Hamburg's red-light district, that appeared in the German magazine *Stern* (June 8, 1978): 'You experience the masculine dream, as seductive as it is absurd, of being coddled by women like a baby and at the same time commanding them like a pascha.' This 'dream' is in fact not absurd; it arises from the infant's most genuine and legitimate needs. Our world would be very different if the majority of babies had the chance to rule over their mothers like paschas and to be coddled by them, without having to concern themselves with their mothers' needs.

The reporter asked some of the regular clients what gave them most pleasure in these establishments and summarized their answers as follows:

> that the girls are available and completely at the customer's disposal; they do *not require protestations of love like girlfriends*. There are *no obligations, psychological dramas,* or *pangs of conscience* when desire has passed: 'You pay and are free!' Even (and especially) the *humiliation* that such an encounter also involves for the client can *increase stimulation* – but that is less willingly mentioned.*

*Italics added.

The humiliation, self-disgust, and self-contempt trigger the past situation and, through the compulsion to repeat, produce the same tragic conditions for pleasure. Seen in this way, the compulsion to repeat is a great opportunity. It can be resolved when the feelings in the present situation can be felt and clarified. If no use is made of this opportunity, if its message is ignored, the compulsion to repeat will continue without abating for the person's entire lifetime, although its form may change.

What is unconscious cannot be abolished by proclamation or prohibition. One can, however, develop sensitivity toward recognizing it and begin to experience it consciously, and thus eventually gain control over it. A mother cannot truly respect her child as long as she does not realize what deep shame she causes him with an ironic remark, intended only to cover her own uncertainty. Indeed, she cannot be aware of how deeply humiliated, despised, and devalued her child feels, if she herself has never consciously suffered these feelings, and if she tries to fend them off with irony.

The same can be said for most psychiatrists, clinical psychologists, and therapists. Certainly, they do not use words like 'bad,' 'dirty,' 'naughty,' 'egoistic,' 'rotten' – but among themselves they sometimes speak of 'narcissistic,' 'exhibitionistic,' 'destructive,' 'regressive,' or 'borderline' patients without noticing that they give these words a pejorative meaning. It may be that their abstract vocabulary, their supposedly objective attitudes, even the way they formulate their theories and zealously make their diagnoses, all have something in common with a mother's contemptuous looks – which they could, if they were willing, trace to the accommodating three-year-old girl or boy within themselves.

It is understandable that a patient's scornful attitude could induce a therapist to protect his superiority with the help of theory. But if he builds such a wall, the patient's true self will not be visible to him. It will hide from him just as it did from the mother's disgusted eyes. We could, however, make good use of our sensitivity by instead detecting pieces of the story of a despised child that lie behind all the patient's expressions of contempt. When the therapist's resources are used in this way, it is easier for him not to feel he is being attacked and to drop his need to hide behind his theories. Knowledge of theory is essential, but knowledge of the theory must not have a defensive function: It must not become the successor of a strict, controlling mother, forcing the therapist to accommodate himself to it.

'DEPRAVITY' AS 'EVIL' IN HERMANN HESSE'S CHILDHOOD WORLD

It is very difficult to describe how people deal with the contempt under which they suffered as children –

especially the contempt for all their sensual enjoyment and pleasure in living – without giving concrete examples. With the aid of theoretical models, I could certainly describe the various defense mechanisms, especially the defense against feelings, but doing so would fail to communicate the emotional climate, which alone evokes a person's suffering and so makes identification and empathy possible for the reader. With purely theoretical representations, we therapists remain 'outside'; from there we can talk about the 'others,' classify, group, and label them by making diagnoses, and discuss them in a language only we understand. If we refuse to do all that, we need examples. It is only through the details of a specific life that we can show how a person has experienced the naughtiness of his childhood as 'wickedness itself.' Only the history of an individual life can make us realize how impossible it is for a child to recognize his parents' compulsions as such and to realize that this blindness can persist throughout the adult's whole life, try as he may to break out of his inner prison.

I use the example of the poet and novelist Hermann Hesse to demonstrate this very complicated situation. This example has the advantage of having been published, and published by the person himself, so that the connections that I postulate can be clarified with concrete examples from his life.

At the beginning of his novel *Demian*, Hermann

Hesse describes the 'goodness and purity' of a parental home in which there is no room for a child's fibs. (It is not difficult to recognize the author's own parental home in this novel, and he confirms this indirectly.) The child is alone with his sin and feels that he is depraved, wicked, and outcast, through nobody scolds him, since no one as yet knows the 'terrible facts.' This situation is of course a common one in real life, and Hesse's idealized way of describing such a 'pure' household is not strange to us either. It reflects both the child's point of view and the hidden cruelty of commonplace methods, with which we are only too familiar, used to teach moral 'values.'

Like most parents [writes Hesse], mine were no help with the new problems of puberty, to which no reference was ever made. All they did was take *endless trouble* in supporting my hopeless attempts to *deny reality* and to continue dwelling in a childhood world that was becoming *more and more unreal*. I have no idea whether parents can be of help, and I do not blame mine. It was my own affair to come to terms with myself and to find my own way, and like most well-brought-up children, I managed it badly. (p. 49)*

*Italics added.

The Drama of Being a Child

A child's parents seem to him to be free of sexual desires, for they have means and possibilities of hiding their sexual activities, whereas the child is always under surveillance.* The first part of *Demian*, it seems to me, is very evocative and easy to appreciate, even for people from quite different milieus. What makes the later parts of the novel so peculiarly difficult must in some way be related to Hesse's parents' and grandparents' moral values (they were missionary families). These permeate many of his stories but can perhaps be most easily sensed in *Demian*.

Although Sinclair, the hero, has already had his own experience of cruelty (blackmail by an older boy), it has given him no key to a better understanding of the world. 'Wickedness' for him is 'depravity' (here is the missionaries' language): it is neither hate nor cruelty, but such trivialities as drinking in a tavern.

As a little boy, Hermann Hesse took over from his parents this particular concept of wickedness as depravity. It is like a foreign body that he seeks to locate and

*In his story 'A Child's Heart,' Hesse writes: 'The adults acted as if the world were perfect and as if they themselves were demigods, we children were nothing but scum. . . . Again and again, after a few days, even after a few hours, something happened that should not have been allowed, something wretched, depressing, and shaming. Again and again, in the midst of the noblest and staunchest decisions and vows, I fell abruptly, inescapably, into sin and wickedness, into ordinary bad habits. Why was it this way?' (pp. 7, 8)

112

uproot from his personality. This is why everything that happens in *Demian* after the appearance of the god Abraxas, who is to 'unite the godly and the devilish,' is so curiously removed. Wickedness is supposed to be artfully united with goodness here, but we are not touched by it. One has the impression that, for the boy, this is something strange, threatening, and above all unknown, from which he nevertheless cannot free himself. His emotional belief in 'depravity' is already joined to fear and guilt:

> Once more I was trying most strenuously to con-
> struct an intimate 'world of light' for myself out of
> the shambles of a period of devastation; once
> more I sacrificed everything within me to the aim
> of banishing darkness and evil from myself. (pp.
> 81–82)

In the Zürich exhibition (1977) to commemorate the centennial of Hesse's birth, a picture was displayed that had hung above the little Hermann's bed and that he had grown up with. In this picture, on the right, we see the 'good' road to heaven, full of thorns, difficulties, and suffering. On the left, we see the easy, pleasurable road that inevitably leads to hell. Taverns play a prominent part on this road, probably because devout women hoped to keep their husbands and sons away from these wicked places with this threatening representation. These taverns play an important role in *Demian* – ironically so, because Hesse had no urge at all to get drunk in such taverns, though he certainly did wish to break out of the narrowness of his parents' values.

Every child forms his first image of what is 'bad' quite concretely, by what is forbidden – by his parents' prohibitions, taboos, and fears. He will have a long way to go before he can free himself from these parental values and see without filters what he has believed to be 'badness' in himself. He will then no longer regard it as 'depraved' and 'wicked,' but as a comprehensible latent reaction to injuries he had to repress when a child. As an adult, he can discover the causes and free himself from this unconscious reaction. He also has the opportunity to apologize for what he has done to others out of ignorance, blindness, and confusion, and doing so will help him to avoid repetitions of acts he no longer wishes to continue.

Unfortunately, the path to clarification was not open to Hermann Hesse. The following passage from *Demian* shows how deeply the perceived loss of his parents' love threatened his search for his true self:

But where we have given of our love and respect not from habit but of our own free will, where we have been disciples and friends out of our inmost hearts, it is a bitter and horrible moment when we

114

suddenly recognize that the current within us wants to pull us away from what is dearest to us. Then every thought that rejects the friend and mentor turns on our own hearts like a *poisoned barb*, then each blow struck in defense *flies back into one's own face*, the words 'disloyalty' and 'ingratitude' strike the person who feels he was morally sound *like catcalls and stigma*, and the *frightened heart flees timidly back* to the *charmed valleys of childhood* virtues, unable to believe that this break, too, must be made, this bond also broken. (p. 127)*

And in his story 'A Child's Heart' we read:

If I were to reduce all my feelings and their painful conflicts to a single name, I can think of no other word but: dread. It was dread, dread and uncertainty, that I felt in all those hours of shattered childhood felicity: dread of punishment, dread of my own conscience, dread of stirrings in my soul which I considered forbidden and criminal. (p. 10)

In this story Hesse portrays with great tenderness and understanding the feelings of an eleven-year-old

*Italics added.

115

boy who has stolen some dried figs from his beloved father's room so that he could have in his possession something that belongs to his father. Guilt feelings, fear, and despair torment him in his loneliness and are replaced at last by the deepest humiliation and shame when his 'wicked deed' is discovered. The strength of this portrayal leads us to surmise that it concerns a real episode from Hesse's own childhood. This surmise becomes certainty, thanks to a note made by his mother on November 11, 1889: 'Hermann's theft of figs discovered.'

From the entries in his mother's diary and from the extensive exchange of letters between both parents and various members of the family, which have been available since 1966, it is possible to guess at the small boy's painful path. Hesse, like so many gifted children, was so difficult for his parents to bear not despite but *because of* his inner riches. Often a child's very gifts (his great intensity of feeling, depth of experience, curiosity, intelligence, quickness – and his ability to be critical) will confront his parents with conflicts that they have long sought to keep at bay by means of rules and regulations. These regulations must then be rescued at the cost of the child's development. All this can lead to an apparently paradoxical situation when parents who are proud of their gifted child and who even admire him are forced by their own repression to reject, suppress, or even destroy what is *best*, because truest, in that child. Two of Hesse's mother's observations may illustrate how this work of destruction can be combined with apparent loving care:

1: (1881): 'Hermann is going to nursery school, his violent temperament causes us much distress.' (1966, p. 10) The child was three years old.

2: (1884): 'Things are going better with Hermann, whose education causes us so much distress and trouble. From the 21st of January to the 5th of June he lived wholly in the boys' house and only spent Sundays with us. He behaved well there but came home pale, thin and *depressed*. The *effects are decidedly good and salutary*. He is much *easier to manage now*.' (1966, pp. 13-14) The child now was seven years old.*

On November 14, 1883, his father, Johannes Hesse, wrote:

Hermann, who was considered almost a model of good behavior in the boys' house is sometimes *hardly to be borne*. Though it would be very humiliating *for us*[!], I am earnestly considering whether we should not place him in an *institution or another household*. We are too nervous and weak for him, and the whole household [is] too undisciplined and irregular. He seems to be gifted for everything: he observes the moon and the clouds,

*Italics added.

117

extemporizes for long periods on the harmonium, draws wonderful pictures with pencil or pen, can sing quite well when he wants to, and is never at a loss for a rhyme.*(1966, p. 13)

In the strongly idealized picture of his childhood and his parents that we encounter in *Hermann Lauscher*,[†] Hesse has completely abandoned the original, rebellious, 'difficult,' and – for his parents – troublesome child he once was. He had no way to accommodate this important part of his self and so was forced to expel it. Perhaps this is why his great and genuine longing for his true self remained unfulfilled.

That Hermann Hesse was not deficient in courage, talent, or depth of feeling is, of course, evident in his works and in many of his letters, especially the outraged letter from the institution in Stetten. But his father's answer to this letter (see Hesse, 1966), his

---

*Italics added.

†When my childhood at times stirs my heart, it is like a gold-framed, deep-toned picture in which predominates a wealth of chestnuts and alders, an indescribably delightful morning light and a background of splendid mountains. All the hours in my life, in which I was allowed a short period of peace, forgetful of the world; all the lonely walks, which I took over beautiful mountains; all the moments in which an unexpected happiness, or love without desire, carried me away from yesterday and tomorrow; all these can be given no more precious name than when I compared them with this green picture of my earliest life.' (*Gesammelte Werke*, vol. I, Frankfurt: M. Suhrkamp, 1970, p. 218)

mother's notes, and the passages from *Demian* and 'A
Child's Heart' quoted above show us clearly how the
crushing weight of the denial of his childhood pain
pressed on him. Despite his enormous acclaim and
success, and despite the Nobel Prize, Hesse in his
mature years suffered from the tragic and painful state
of being separated from his true self, to which doctors
refer offhandedly as depression.

THE MOTHER AS SOCIETY'S AGENT DURING THE FIRST
YEARS OF LIFE

If we were to tell a patient that in other societies his
perversion would not be a problem, that it is a problem
here only because it is our society that is sick and produces constrictions and constraints, we would certainly
be telling him at least a partial truth, but it would be of
little help to him. He would feel, rather, that as an individual, with his own individual history, he was being
passed over and misunderstood, for this interpretation
makes too little of his own very real tragedy. What he
most needs to understand is his compulsion to repeat,
and the state of affairs behind it to which this compulsion bears witness. His plight is no doubt the result of
social pressures, but these do not have their effect on
his psyche through abstract knowledge; they are firmly
anchored in his earliest affective experience with his
mother. Thus his problems cannot be solved with

words, but only through *experience* – not merely corrective experience as an adult but, above all, through a conscious experience of his early fear of his beloved mother's contempt and his subsequent feelings of indignation and sadness. Mere words, however skilled the interpretation, will leave unchanged or even deepen the split between intellectual speculation and the knowledge of the body, the split from which he already suffers.

One can therefore hardly free an addict from the cruelty of his addiction by showing him how the absurdity, exploitation, and perversity of society cause our neuroses and perversions, however true this may be. The addict will love such explanations and eagerly believe them, because they spare him the pain of the truth. But things we can see through do not make us sick, although they may arouse our indignation, anger, sadness, or feelings of impotence. What makes us sick are those things we cannot see through, society's constraints that we have absorbed through our parents' eyes. No amount of reading or learning can free us from those eyes.

To put it another way: Many people suffering from severe symptoms are very intelligent. They read in newspapers and books about the absurdity of the arms race, about exploitation through capitalism, diplomatic insincerity, the arrogance and manipulation of power, submission of the weak, and the impotence of individuals – and they have given thought to these subjects. What they do not see, because they cannot see them, are the absurdities enacted by their own mothers when they were still tiny children.

Oppression and the forcing of submission do not begin in the office, factory, or political party; they begin in the very first weeks of an infant's life. Afterward they are repressed and are then, because of their very nature, inaccessible to argument. Nothing changes in the character of submission or dependency, when it is only their object that is changed.

Political action can be fed by the unconscious rage of children who have been misused, imprisoned, exploited, cramped, and drilled. This rage can be partially discharged in fighting 'enemies,' without having to give up the idealization of one's own parents. The old dependency will then simply be shifted to a new group or leader. If, however, disillusionment and the resultant mourning can be lived through, social and political disengagement do not usually follow, but our actions are freed from the compulsion to repeat. They can then have a clear goal, formed out of conscious decisions.

Once our own reality has been faced and experienced, the inner necessity to keep building up new illusions and denials in order to avoid the experience of that reality disappears. We then realize that all our lives we have feared and struggled to ward off something that really cannot happen any longer; it has already happened, at the very beginning of our lives while we were completely dependent.

Therapeutic effects (in the form of temporary improvement) may be achieved if a strict conscience can be replaced by the therapist's or the group's more tolerant one. The aim of therapy, however, is not to correct the past, but to enable the patient both to confront his own history and to grieve over it. The patient has to discover early memories within himself and must become consciously aware of his parents' unconscious manipulation and contempt, so that he can free himself from them. As long as he has to make do with a substitute tolerance, borrowed from his therapist or his group, the contemptuous attitudes he inherited from his parents will remain hidden in his unconscious, unchanged despite all his improved intellectual knowledge and intentions. This contemptuous attitude will show itself in the patient's human relationships and will continue to torment him as long as it functions in the cells of his body. The contents of the unconscious remain unchanged and timeless. It is only as these contents become conscious that change can begin.

THE LONELINESS OF THE CONTEMPTUOUS

The contempt shown by many disturbed people may have various forerunners in their life history, but the function all expressions of contempt have in common is the defense against unwanted feelings. Contempt simply evaporates, having lost its point, when it is no longer useful as a shield – against the child's shame over his desperate, unreturned love; against his feeling of inadequacy; or above all against his rage that his parents were not available. Once we are able to feel and understand the repressed emotions of childhood, we will no longer need contempt as a defense against them. On the other hand, as long as we despise the other person and over-value our own achievements ('he can't do what I can do'), we do not have to mourn the fact that love is not forthcoming without achievement. Nevertheless, if we avoid this mourning it means that we remain at bottom the one who is despised, for we have to despise everything in ourselves that is not wonderful, good, and clever. Thus we perpetuate the loneliness of childhood: We despise weakness, helplessness, uncertainty – in short, the child in ourselves and in others.

The contempt for others in grandiose, successful people always includes disrespect for their own true selves, as their scorn implies: 'Without these superior qualities of mine, a person is completely worthless.' This means further: 'Without these achievements, these gifts, I could never be loved, would never have been loved.' Grandiosity in the adult guarantees that the illusion continues: 'I was loved.' The way out of this confusing and stressful self-betrayal may well be illustrated by John's dream.

John, forty-eight, who came back to therapy because of tormenting obsessions, repeatedly dreamed that he was on a lookout tower that stood in a swampy area at the edge of a town dear to him. In reality, the town had no such tower, but it belonged unequivocally to John's dream landscape, and he knew it well. From there he had a lovely view, but he felt sad and deserted. There was an elevator in the tower, and in the dream there were all kinds of difficulties over entrance tickets and obstacles on the way to this tower. The dream recurred often, with the same feelings of being deserted.

Only after much had changed in the course of therapy were there new variations in the dream, too, and at last it changed in a decisive way. John was first surprised to dream that he already had entrance tickets, but the tower had been demolished and there was no longer a view. Instead, he saw a bridge that joined the swampy district to the town. He could thus go on foot into the town and see 'not everything' but 'some things close up.' John, who suffered from an elevator phobia, was somewhat relieved, for he had felt considerable anxiety riding in this elevator. Speaking of the dream, he said he was perhaps no longer dependent on always having a complete view, on always seeing everything – being on top and cleverer than other people. He now could go on foot like everyone else.

John was the more astonished when he later dreamed that he was suddenly sitting in this elevator in the tower again and was being drawn upward as in a chair lift, without feeling any fear. He enjoyed the ride, got out at the top, and, strange to say, found colorful life all about him. He was on a plateau, from where he had a view of the valleys. There was also a town up there, with a bazaar full of colorful wares; a school where children were practicing ballet and he could join in (this had been a childhood wish); and groups of people holding discussions, with whom he sat and talked. He felt integrated into this society, just as he was. Although the dream expressed his wishes rather than reality, it showed him his true, *real* needs: to be loved and to love beyond his achievements. This dream impressed him deeply. He said:

My earlier dreams of the tower showed my isolation and loneliness. At home, as the eldest, I was always ahead of my siblings, my parents could not match my intelligence, and in all intellectual matters I was alone. On the one hand, I had to demonstrate my knowledge in order to be taken seriously, and on the other, I had to hide it or my parents would say: 'Your studies are going to your head! Do you think you are better than everyone else, just because you had the chance to study? Without your mother's sacrifice and your father's hard work you would never have been able to do it.' That made me feel guilty and I tried to hide my difference, my interests, and my gifts. I wanted to be like the others. There was no way for me to be true to myself, to respect me as I really was.

So John had searched for his tower and had struggled with obstacles (on the way, with entrance tickets, his fears, and more), and when he got to the top – that is, was smarter than the others – he felt lonely and deserted.

It is a well-known and common paradox that parents who take up this grudging and competitive attitude toward their child at the same time urge him on to the greatest achievement and are proud of his success. Thus John *had to* look for his tower and had to encounter obstacles, as well. Eventually he went through a revolt against this pressure toward achievement and stress, and so the tower disappeared in the first of the dreams I have described here. He could give up his grandiose fantasy of seeing *everything* from above and could look at things in his beloved town (in himself) from close by.

Only now did it become clear to him that he had felt compelled to isolate himself from others by means of his contempt and at the same time was isolated and separated from his true self – at least from its helpless, uncertain part.

The Vicious Circle of Contempt

Contempt as a rule will cease with the beginning of mourning for the irreversible that cannot be changed, for contempt, too, has in its own way served to deny the reality of the past. It is, after all, less painful to think that the others do not understand because they are too stupid. Then one can make efforts to explain things to them, and the illusion of being understood ('if only I can express myself properly') can be maintained.* If, however, this effort is relaxed, one is forced to realize that understanding was not possible, since the repression of the parents' own childhood needs made them blind to their children's needs.

Even alert parents cannot always understand their children, but they will respect their children's feelings even when they cannot understand them. Where there is no such respect, their children seek refuge from a painful truth in ideologies. Nationalism, racism, and fascism are in fact nothing other than ideological guises of the flight from painful, unconscious memories of endured contempt into the dangerous, destructive disrespect for human life, glorified as a political program. The formerly hidden cruelty that was exercised upon the powerless child now becomes only too apparent in the violence of such 'political' groups. Its origins in

---

*Devastating examples of this process are the works of van Gogh (see Nagara, 1967), who so wonderfully and so unsuccessfully courted the favor of his mother with all the means at his disposal.

childhood, in the total disregard of the former child, however, remain concealed or absolutely denied, not only by the members of these groups but by society as a whole.

ACHIEVING FREEDOM FROM CONTEMPT AND
RESPECTING LIFE

Sexual perversions, obsessions, and flights into ideologies are not the only possibilities for perpetuating the tragedy of early suffering from contempt. There are countless ways we may transmit the family climate under which we suffered as children. There are people, for example, who never say a loud or angry word, who seem to be only good and noble, and who still give others the palpable feeling of being ridiculous or stupid or too noisy, or at any rate too common compared with themselves. They do not know it and perhaps do not intend it, but this is what they radiate: the attitude of their parents, of which they have never been aware. The children of such persons find it particularly difficult to formulate any reproach until they learn to do so in their therapy.

Then there are the people who can seem very friendly, if a shade patronizing, but in whose presence one feels as if one were nothing. They convey the feeling that they are the only ones who exist, the only ones who have anything interesting or relevant to say. The

others can only stand there and admire them in fascination, or turn away in disappointment and sorrow
about their own lack of worth, unable to express themselves in these persons' presence. These people might
be the children of grandiose parents, whom they as
children had no hope of emulating; but later, as adults,
they unconsciously pass on this atmosphere to those
around them.

Quite a different impression will be given by those
people who, as children, were intellectually far beyond
their parents and therefore admired by them, but who
also therefore had to solve their own problems alone.
These people, who give us a feeling of their intellectual
strength and will power, also seem to demand that we,
too, ought to fight off any feeling of weakness with
intellectual means. In their presence one feels one can't
be recognized as a person with problems – just as they
and their problems were unrecognized by their parents, for whom they always had to be strong.

Keeping these examples in mind, it is easy to see
why some professors or writers who are quite capable
of expressing themselves clearly will use language that
is so convoluted and arcane that their students or readers must struggle angrily to acquire ideas that they then
can make little use of. The students may well experience feelings similar to those their teacher was once
forced to suppress in relation to his parents. If the students themselves become teachers one day, they will

then have the opportunity to hand on this unusable knowledge like a priceless jewel (because it has cost them so much).

It greatly aids the success of therapeutic work when we become aware of our parents' destructive patterns at work within us. But to free ourselves from these patterns we need more than an intellectual awareness: we need an emotional confrontation with our parents in an inner dialogue.

When the patient has emotionally worked through the history of her childhood and has thus regained her sense of being alive, the goal of therapy has been reached. She will then be able to use the tools she has learned whenever feelings from her past are triggered by present events. As time goes on, she will use them more and more effectively and will need less time for this work. The 'map' of her life will be available for her whenever she needs it.

The therapist must leave it up to the patient to decide whether she will take a regular job or not; whether she wants to live alone or with a partner; whether she wants to join a political party, and if so, which one. All of these decisions must be her own. Her life story, her experiences, and what she has learned from them will all play a role in how she will live. It is not the task of the therapist to 'socialize' her, or to 'raise her consciousness' (not even politically, for every form of indoctrination denies her autonomy), or to 'make friendships possible for her.' All that is her own affair.

When the patient has consciously and repeatedly experienced how the whole process of her upbringing manipulated and damaged her in her childhood, and with what desires for revenge this has left her, then she will see through manipulation more quickly than before and will herself have less need to manipulate others. Such a patient will be able to join groups if she wishes without again becoming helplessly dependent or bound, for she has consciously gone through the helplessness and dependency of her childhood. She will be in less danger of idealizing people or systems or being deceived by a guru in a sect if she has realized clearly how as a child she took every word uttered by her mother or father for the deepest wisdom. She may momentarily experience, while listening to a lecture or reading a book, the same old childish fascination and admiration, but she will sooner recognize and reject the underlying emptiness that lurks behind these manipulative and seductive words. A person who has matured through her own experience cannot be tricked with fascinating, incomprehensible words. Finally, a person who has consciously worked through the whole tragedy of her own fate will recognize another's suffering more clearly, though the other may be trying to hide it. She will not be scornful of others' feelings, whatever their nature, because she takes her own feelings seriously and knows how to work with them. She surely will not keep the vicious circle of contempt turning.

This achievement will have not only personal consequences for the individual and her family, but also far-reaching significance for society as a whole. People who discover their past with the help of their feelings, who learn through therapy to clarify these feelings, to look for their *real causes*, and to resolve the transference, will no longer be compelled to displace their hatred onto innocents in order to protect those who have in fact earned this hatred. They will be capable of hating what is hateful and of loving what deserves love. Once they dare to see who brought them to their plight and how it was done, they will be better oriented in present reality and able to avoid acting blindly, unconsciously. They will no longer behave like the mistreated children they were, children who must protect their parents and who therefore need a scapegoat for the buried emotions that torment them.

The future of democracy and democratic freedom depends on our capacity to take this very step and to recognize that it is simply impossible to struggle successfully against hatred outside ourselves, while ignoring its messages within. We must know and use the tools that are necessary to resolve it: We must feel and understand its source and its legitimacy. There is no point in appealing to our goodwill, our kindness, and a common spirit of love, as long as the path to clarifying our feelings is blocked by the unconscious fear of our parents.

Consciously experiencing our legitimate emotions is liberating, not just because of the discharge of long-held tensions in the body but above all because it opens our eyes to reality (both past and present) and frees us of lies and illusions. It gives us back repressed memories and helps dispel attendant symptoms. It is therefore empowering without being destructive. Repressed emotion can be resolved as soon as it is felt, understood, and recognized as legitimate. Being detached from it becomes possible and this is totally different from repression.

But illegitimate hatred never disappears. It may switch scapegoats, but it will remain ever-present and undiluted. It cannot be appeased: It poisons and blinds the soul, devours the memory and the mind, and kills the capacity for compassion and insight. Its destructive power stems from a history of horror that has been repressed and stored in the body but that, without effective therapy, has no direct access to the conscious mind. Hating and offending an innocent person, using him as a scapegoat, can only strengthen the walls of our inner prison of confusion, isolation, fear, and loneliness; it cannot free us. A house built out of self-betrayal will sooner or later fall down and mercilessly destroy human life – if not that of the builder, then that of his children, who will sense the lie without being aware of it and who will end up paying the full price for this hidden arrangement.

A person who can honestly and without self-deception deal with his feelings has no need to disguise them with the help of ideologies. The basic similarity of the various nationalistic movements flourishing today reveals that their motives have nothing to do with the real interests of the people who are fighting and hating, but instead have very much to do with those people's childhood histories. The mistreatment, humiliation, and exploitation of children is the same worldwide, as is the means of avoiding the memory of it. Individuals who do not want to know their own truth collude in denial with society as a whole, looking for a common 'enemy' on whom to act out their repressed rage. But as the inhabitants of this shrinking planet near the end of the twentieth century, the danger inherent in self-deception is growing exponentially – and we can afford it less than ever. Fortunately, at the same time, we now have the tools we need to truly understand ourselves, as we were and as we are.

Afterword for the 2007 Edition

This book was first published almost 30 years ago. Even now, readers tell me that it brought into their lives the tormented, isolated, never-understood child within them whom they had forgotten and abandoned decades before. Many say that for the first time in their lives, they can feel the plight of this child and can cry about the pain of their childhood, of which they were not truly aware for such a long time. They often say, 'You described my life and my family,' and they ask, 'How did you know them?'

The strong emotional impact of this book may come from the fact that writing it brought about my own emotional awakening. It came with my decision to find my own history, to live my own life, and to leave behind me everything I felt was not actually ME, was only the product of my upbringing.

A decision like this initiates a process that needs time. I am happy now that I have used this time (almost 30 years) to become more and more free from conventional ways of thinking and from theories that were built to conceal and obscure the reality of childhood: the extraordinary pain we were exposed to and the necessity to repress our feelings into our bodies, our unconsciousness, in order to survive.

With this insight began the story of my research that included the childhood stories of dictators and famous writers who died very early. In all these cases I found without any exceptions the same patterns: the denial of the once endured terror, the idolizing of the extremely abusive parents, and a destructive or self-destructive behavior as a result.

My exploration of this reality found its expression in all my books, especially in the latest ones, *The Body Never Lies* and *Your Saved Life* (not yet translated into English). Also, articles and interviews on my Web site can provide the recent readers of *Drama* with many conclusions to which my research on childhood brought me in the last ten years.

But above all, my answers to readers' mail can illustrate the concept of therapy that I developed in the last several years. In addition, many letters on the Web site show how people succeeded in overcoming their physical symptoms by facing the stories of their childhood, feeling their indignation, liberating themselves from their destructive self-blame, and becoming less and less dependent on their abusive parents. This encourages others to feel what they have tried to avoid their whole lives, and it demonstrates that these efforts are effective, that they often help to overcome even chronic illnesses, and that they are not at all dangerous. The once-beaten children still living inside adults often fear being punished if they dare to truly SEE, without illusions, what their parents did to them in their first years of life. Once they understand that this danger no longer exists, they can liberate their life.

I assume that the Web site gives answers to the questions this book raises, but without reading it, without making this step, without opening the door to the child you once were, the full impact of the Web site may be missed. The child you have found by reading *Drama* will hopefully lead you to read the material on the Web site, to find the information you may need today and to benefit from it.

Alice Miller
2007

Works Cited

Eicke-Spengler, M. 1977. Zur Entwicklung der Theorie der Depression. *Psyche* 31:1077–1125.

Ganz, H. 1966. *Pestalozzi*. Zurich: Origo.

Hesse, H. 1965. *Demian*. New York: Harper & Row; London: Peter Owen.

————. 1970. *Gesammelte Werke*. Frankfurt: M. Suhrkamp.

————. 1966. 'Kindheit und Jugend vor Neunzehnhundert.' In *Briefen und Lebenszeugnissen 1877–1895*. Frankfurt: M. Suhrkamp.

————. 1971. 'A child's heart.' In *Klingsor's last summer*. New York: Harper & Row; London: Jonathan Cape.

Jenson, J. 1995 *Reclaiming Your Life: A step-by-step guide to using regression therapy to overcome the effects of child-hood abuse.* New York: Dutton.

Lavater-Sloman, M. 1977. *Pestalozzi*. Zurich and Munich: Artemis.

Miller, A. 1983. *For your own good: The roots of violence in child-rearing.* New York: Farrar, Straus and Giroux; London: Virago Press.

————. 1984. *Thou shalt not be aware: Society's betrayal of the child.* New York: Farrar, Straus and Giroux, (PB) New American Library; London: Pluto Press.

————. 1986. *Pictures of a childhood: 66 watercolors and an essay.* New York: Farrar, Straus and Giroux. (PB) Meridian/Penguin; London: Virago Press (1995, with a new preface).

————. 1990a. *The untouched key: Tracing childhood trauma in creativity and destructiveness.* New York: Doubleday, (PB) Anchor Press; London: Virago Press.

————. 1990b. *Banished knowledge: Facing childhood injuries.* New York: Doubleday, (PB) Anchor Press; London: Virago Press.

————. 1993. *Breaking down the wall of silence: To join the waiting child.* (PB with an essay). New York: Meridian/Penguin; London: Virago Press.

Mueller-Braunschweig, H. 1974. Psychopathologie und Kreativität. *Psyche* 28: 600–654.

Nagara, H. 1967. *Vincent van Gogh.* London: Allen and Unwin.

Appendix

To preserve the associative style of the original *Drama* and keep its contents accessible to the lay reader, I have tried not to overload this book with references. Interested professionals can, however, refer for specific topics to the books I have written in the years since the *Drama* was first published:

1. The issue of *manipulation in therapy* is dealt with extensively in *Thou Shalt Not Be Aware*, with specific references to various therapy techniques which I consider to be manipulative.

2. The issue of *manipulation and mistreatment in childhood* is the main theme of F*or Your Own Good*, where I also substantiate, with well-known examples, my opinion on the roots of serial crimes, murder, and drug addiction.

3. The goal of the revised version of the *Drama* is above all to make people aware of the fact that it is impossible either to receive or to provide real therapeutic help as long as the personal, emotional confrontation with one's own past is avoided. As the tendency to escape the truth of one's unique history by means of theoretical, religious, pseudo-scientific, and (always) manipulative concepts continues to be very fashionable, I wanted to be as clear as possible on this point. I hope that my rather broad descriptions of certain 'therapies' and the readers' own experience with

self-therapy will make them more alert and better able to recognize these misleading concepts on their own, should they be exposed to them in the future.

Appendix

This is a text I wrote in 1984 that has appeared frequently in newspapers. I include it here because it may prove helpful to the reader who has not read my earlier books.

In 1613, when Galileo Galilei presented mathematical proof for the Copernican theory that the Earth revolves around the Sun and not the opposite, it was labeled 'false and absurd' by the Church. Galileo was forced to recant, and, perhaps as a result, subsequently became blind. Not until three hundred years later did the Church finally decide to give up its illusion and remove his writings from the Index.

Now we find ourselves in a situation similar to that of the Church in Galileo's time, but for us today much more hangs in the balance. Whether we decide for truth or illusion will have far more serious consequences for the survival of humanity than was the case in the seventeenth century. For some years now, there has been evidence that the devastating effects of the traumatization of children take their toll on society, leading to inconceivable violence in society and to the repetition of child abuse in the next generation – a phenomenon that we are still forbidden to recognize. This knowledge concerns every single one of us and – if disseminated widely enough – should lead to fundamental changes in society, above all to a halt in the blind escalation of violence. The following points are intended to amplify my meaning:

1. All children are born to grow, to develop, to live, to love, and to articulate their needs and feelings for their self-protection.

2. For their development, children need the respect and protection of adults who take them seriously, love them, and honestly help them to become oriented in the world.

3. When these vital needs are frustrated and children are, instead, abused for the sake of adults' needs by being exploited, beaten, punished, taken advantage of, manipulated, neglected, or deceived without the intervention of any witness, then their integrity will be lastingly impaired.

4. The normal reactions to such injury should be anger and pain; since children in this hurtful kind of environment, however, are forbidden to express their anger and since it would be unbearable to experience their pain all alone, they are compelled to suppress their feelings, repress all memory of the trauma, and idealize those guilty of the abuse. Later they will have no memory of what was done to them.

5. Disassociated from the original cause, their feelings of anger, helplessness, despair, longing, anxiety, and pain will find expression in destructive acts against others (criminal behavior, mass murder) or against themselves (drug addiction, alcoholism, prostitution, psychic disorders, suicide).

6. If these people become parents, they will often direct acts of revenge for their mistreatment in childhood against their own children, whom they use as scapegoats. Child abuse is still sanctioned – indeed, held in high regard – in our society as long as it is defined as child rearing. It is a tragic fact that parents beat their children in order to escape the emotions stemming from how they were treated by their own parents.

7. If mistreated children are not to become criminals or mentally ill, it is essential that at least once in their life they come in contact with a person who knows without any doubt that the environment, not the helpless, battered child, is at fault. In this regard, knowledge

or ignorance on the part of society can be instrumental in either saving or destroying a life. Here lies the great opportunity for relatives, social workers, therapists, teachers, doctors, psychiatrists, officials, and nurses to support the child and to believe him or her.

8. Till now, society has protected the adult and blamed the victim. It has been abetted in its blindness by theories, still in keeping with pedagogical principles of our great-grandparents, according to which children are viewed as crafty creatures, dominated by wicked drives, who invent stories and attack their innocent parents or desire them sexually. In reality, children tend to blame themselves for their parents' cruelty and to absolve the parents, whom they invariably love, of all responsibility.

9. For some years now, it has been possible to prove, thanks to the use of new therapeutic methods, that repressed traumatic experiences in childhood are stored up in the body and, although remaining unconscious, exert their influence even in adulthood. In addition, electronic testing of the fetus has revealed a fact previously unknown to most adults: A child responds to and learns both tenderness and cruelty from the very beginning.

10. In the light of this new knowledge, even the most absurd behavior reveals its formerly hidden logic once the traumatic experiences of childhood no longer must remain shrouded in darkness.

11. Our sensitization to the cruelty with which children are treated, until now commonly denied, and to the consequences of such treatment will as a matter of course bring to an end the perpetuation of violence from generation to generation.

12. People whose integrity has not been damaged in childhood, who were protected, respected, and treated with honesty by their parents, will be – both in their youth and adulthood – intelligent, responsive, emphatic, and highly sensitive. They will take pleasure in life and will not feel any need to kill or even hurt others or themselves. They will use their power to defend themselves but not to attack others. They will not be able to do otherwise than to respect and protect those weaker than themselves, including their children, because this is what they have learned from their own experience and because it is *this* knowledge (and not the experience of cruelty) that has been stored up inside them from the beginning. Such people will be incapable of understanding why earlier generations had to build up a gigantic war industry in order to feel at ease and safe in this world. Since it will not have to be their unconscious life-task to ward off intimidation experienced at a very early age, they will be able to deal with attempts at intimidation in their adult life more rationally and more creatively.

Index